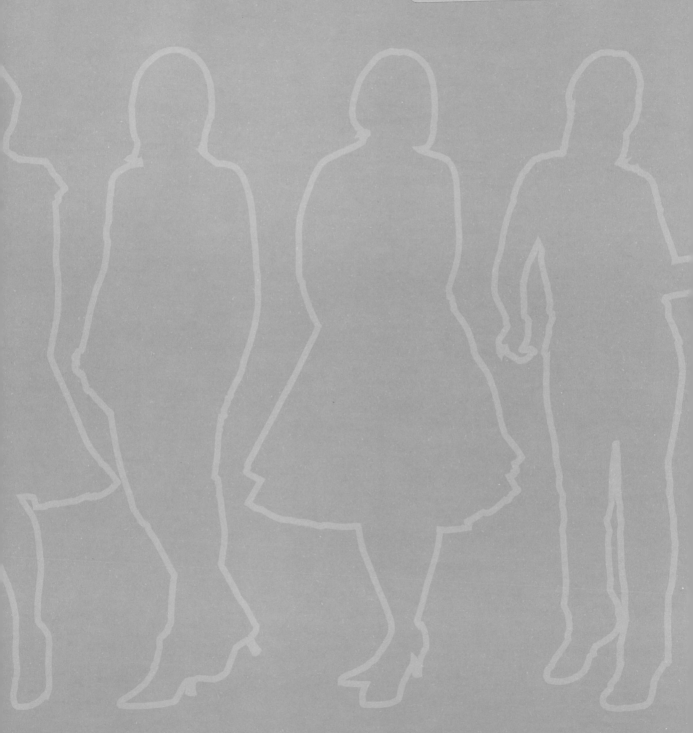

# What to wear when you are losing weight

First published in Great Britain by Simon & Schuster UK Ltd. 2007
A CBS Company

Simon & Schuster UK Ltd
Africa House
64-78 Kingsway
London
WC2B 6AH

1 3 5 7 9 10 8 6 4 2

Design: Andy Summers, Planet Creative
Photography: Ray Moller
Styling: Sharon Agricole
Hair and Make Up: Lisa Collard

Printed and bound in China

ISBN-13: 978–0-774328-578-0
ISBN-10: 0-74328-578-6

With many thanks to the models for this book: Fiona Andreanelli,
Claire Brennan, Lucy Gibbons, Louise Green, Tina Gregory, Aileen King,
Helen Lane, Amanda Shipp, Margaret Simpson. They are all Weight Watcher
Success Stories.

WeightWatchers®

# What to wear when you are losing weight

Vicky Pepys

SIMON &
SCHUSTER

LONDON • NEW YORK • SYDNEY • TORONTO

## About the author

Vicky Pepys is a freelance fashion and style writer. She studied fashion at St Martin's School of Art and assisted Jasper Conran; she's promoted fashionable 'lifestyle' at Lynne Franks PR and learned backstage technique with fashion show producer Mikel Rosen; and there's been a bit of photographic styling in between. She has previously charted her own weight-loss journey (from 17 stone to 12 stone) in a regular column for the *WeightWatchers Magazine*. Vicky currently writes fashion and beauty for *The Journal* daily business paper in Newcastle and is a contributor to *Living North magazine*.

# Contents

# Introduction

Want to change the way you look? Are you at the 'Before' stage and dream of the 'After' look we're all so familiar with in weight-loss magazines?

Weight loss is going to make an incredible difference, sure, but will it suddenly make us stylish? If we dress in dull dark colours and hide under baggy slouchy styles now, who says we will suddenly develop a strong fashion sense when the pounds drop off?

We need to learn some styling secrets as we set off on our weight-loss journey – styling secrets which are as much of an eye-opener as dietary secrets. There are as many fashion blunders as calorie blunders, but as soon as we know about them, we'll never repeat the mistakes.

## Style is a state of mind

What's going to happen to your body in the next few months will be incredible; it's a highly visible physical evolvement and people are going to notice. But how long is it going to take? You know there's no easy answer!

What applies in general is not sure to apply to you – we are all so complex and individual, with different metabolisms, body shapes, appetites and tastes . . . You might as well ask how long is a piece of string. But what can happen

**What's past its sell-by date in the wardrobe isn't going to suddenly recover and revitalise.**

almost immediately is a change in awareness and an experimentation in style. Out with the bad eating habits and out with the bad wardrobe habits at the same time!

Being stylish has nothing to do with a size label – being stylish can begin at whatever size you are now. The latest Health Survey for England (at the time of writing) reveals that at least 45% of women are overweight between the ages of 25–34, 55% are overweight between the ages of 35–44, and 59% are overweight between the ages of 45–54. And the fashion industry is rising (or expanding!) to the occasion. Figures released by TNS Fashion Trak say that approximately £11 billion (at the time of writing) is currently spent on womenswear in the UK and that plus-sizes account for £3.5 billion of it – that's nearly a third of the marketplace. There is more fashion available for size 16 and upwards than ever before. There are stores devoted to plus-sizes, together with internet sites and mail order catalogues. Believe it or not, the larger market is much better catered for than the petite market or the market for the older lady – but stylish petites know how to raid the teen label ranges; and the stylish older lady knows how to experiment with classic shapes and colours, irrespective of labels. So, instead of thinking that trends don't apply to you, the first change that has to be made is a change in your thinking.

We regularly clear our pantry shelves of outdated items that have exceeded their sell-by dates – it's unhealthy to keep these moulding once-edibles. Now we must clear our minds of mouldy old ideas about how we look. And if we can clear our pantry shelves and our minds, why not clear our wardrobes to the same effect? What's past its sell-by date in the wardrobe isn't going to suddenly recover and revitalise. Fresh food equals fresh fashion – both 'go off'. Just as we throw away old food, we must learn to discard clothing that does us no favours.

We know about eating for comfort, it's the same as wearing for comfort – it feels lovely, but it isn't doing us any good at all because we're not looking our best. Our first task is to discard the old and embrace the new, wholeheartedly. The change ahead of us may seem like an awfully long process while we lose a sensible small amount each week, but our wardrobe will really notice every inch.

## How do I begin?

In order to actually begin the change, the starting point is acknowledging that you would like to change. Your reason might be a health concern, an important date in the future where we need to look our best; or just because we don't wish to go on any more as we are. We think being thin will make us more attractive, therefore more successful and an altogether happier human being. We also know this is often hogwash — we can be attractive and happy whatever size we are. But being slimmer might also make us healthier and more physically able. If we're not those things, then we're actually keeping life at bay — and where's the joy in that?

Sometimes the world seems to be made up of only thin and even thinner, doesn't it? Whatever we want to buy seems to be beyond our reach. So at the beginning of this book we will acknowledge and assess what we have, both in our wardrobe, and on our bones, and to some extent within us. We'll learn how to experiment and be daring; we'll develop a whole new attitude of looking at ourselves.

From 'before' to 'after' is an exciting journey: one which maybe we've thought about before, or even attempted to start out on – and just not yet completed. Been here before a couple of times? Then you know the joys of being able to glide on those jeans which wouldn't budge past your hips a couple of months ago; or to wear a skirt with a fixed waistband and a zip, rather than gathered elastic; and to see a graceful neck and shoulder blades emerging. Our physical changes will bring about the determination to reach the final destination for once and for all!

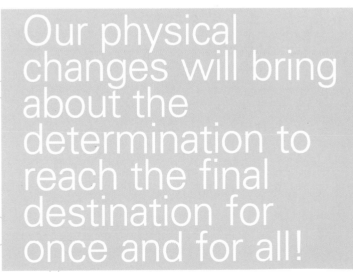

Our physical changes will bring about the determination to reach the final destination for once and for all!

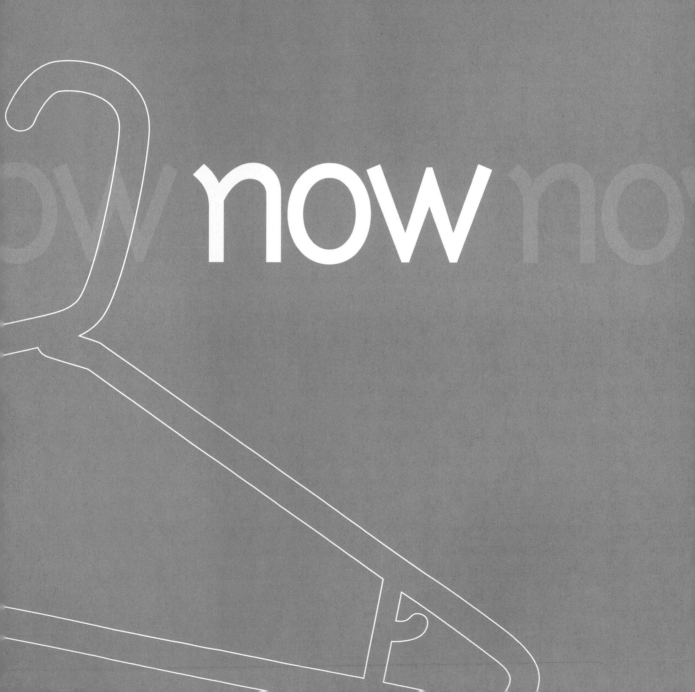

now now now

# Part 1

**Y**ou've bought this book wanting a little bit of help in getting you through the process of dressing fashionably throughout your weight-loss journey. With weight loss comes inch loss, and bang goes most of your existing wardrobe! This is great news, because weight-loss programmes often begin when nothing we like in our wardrobes fits and it's getting increasingly difficult to buy favourite fashion styles. Something's got to give, and it's unlikely to be the seams.

When the first pounds start to drop off and our usual clothes feel a little loose – OK, well, comfortable, like they're supposed to feel – isn't it tempting to 'buy, buy, buy' everything in sight that we can now squeeze into? But we're not made of money, are we? We all have budgets we must adhere to and it's perhaps better to wait for a bit more to drop off, and ultimately reach our target weight, before buying a completely new wardrobe. There are ways of updating an existing wardrobe; it can be tweaked and replaced without splurging all our hard-earned cash on clothes that are an intermediate, short-term answer.

Many of life's problems can be overcome by analysing what's wrong and taking little steps to gradually put things right – rather than trying to hurdle obstacles in difficult giant leaps. So, here we go . . .

The first step is to truly acknowledge our body shape and recognise what we have now, and what we can realistically expect sometime soon, from weight loss. Don't forget that weight-loss programmes bring surprises — even on the weeks when we don't lose pounds, we may lose inches. If you're a previous dieter, you'll know how your body reacts to first weight loss. Where do you lose weight from first?

The most commonly recognised body shapes are 'apple' and 'pear'. Pear-shaped women have a tendency to store fat on the hips, bottom and thighs, but can learn to develop their upper-body strength and develop a better proportion. Apples carry most of their extra pounds around the waist and can find it difficult to lose weight from here. The aim for apples is to look like an eaten core!

Don't worry if you don't fit into either body shape — some of us are a mixture of all sorts! Also some of us may be carrying extra weight, but may have perfect 'hourglass' proportions. We are all so different, thank

> The first step is to acknowledge our body shape and recognise what we have now, and what we can realistically expect sometime soon.

goodness! However, being aware of your body shape, and which body parts you are losing inches from quickest, will help choose flattering clothes.

**FACT**

Are you on this journey because you want to reach goal weight for a special event in the future? Maybe it's a new job, a holiday, a school reunion or a wedding? Start to create a fashion storyboard to keep you going. Tear out pages from magazines of 'perfect' outfits, 'perfect' accessories, the 'perfect' hairdo and the 'perfect' make-up. Keep adding to them and taking away . . . when you've reached your final decisions, they'll be the right ones – and you'll have removed that element of last-minute panic.

## STEP 2 — Size yourself up

A key thing to do is to copy your weight-loss chart from your handbook on to a large sheet of paper and stick it next to your wardrobe, or on the inside of your wardrobe door. Once a week, after your weight-loss meeting, update your chart with the pounds you have lost. Also take your body measurements, to keep track of your inch loss. Add it to your chart.

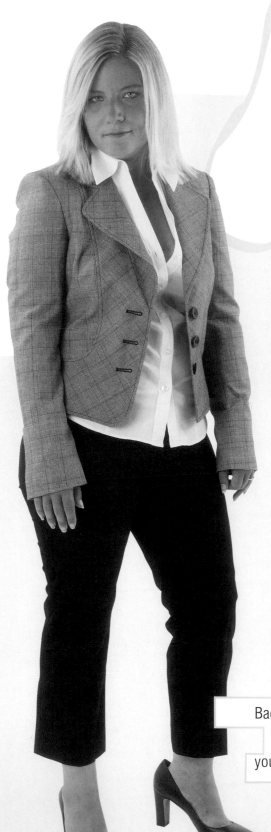

When it comes to choosing garments that are the right size for your changing body shape, you'll need to know four critical measurements: bust, waist, hips, and length (for the individual garment – jacket, sleeve, trouser-leg, dress or skirt). These measurements will help you recognise your size within fashion size ranges and achieve a good and correct fit. Nothing is more unflattering than a garment that fits badly, whatever your shape and size. A jacket-sleeve that's too long can make you look as if you're drowning; a top that's too long can make you look stumpy; Capri-style hipster pants can shorten your legs; and a tight jersey top can make a size 16 look like a 20.

Badly fitting clothes in totally wrong proportions look 'rubbish' whatever your size and shape.

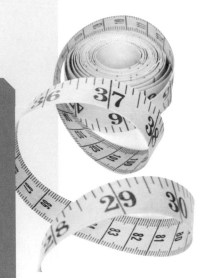

Fashions in general are much bigger these days; for instance, today's size 12 bears no relation to a 1950s' size 12. There are many reasons for this. For instance, we are bigger all over than people in the 1950s because we eat lots of junk food instead of sparse, yet more healthy, wartime rations. And bust sizes are bigger due to underwear design (such as padding) and the popularity of plastic surgery.

## So how do you measure yourself?

Here are some helpful pointers:

✓ Strip down to your bra and pants. You are going to take tight body measurements. Think firm but not squeezed. Note them down in both inches and centimetres.

✓ Measure the fullest part of the bust, making sure that the tape doesn't dip at the back. (This can be quite difficult to do by yourself.)

✓ Measure the natural waist – look for the thinnest part of your body.

✓ Measure the widest part of your hips.

✓ Measure a variety of different lengths depending on the types of garments you're aiming to wear.

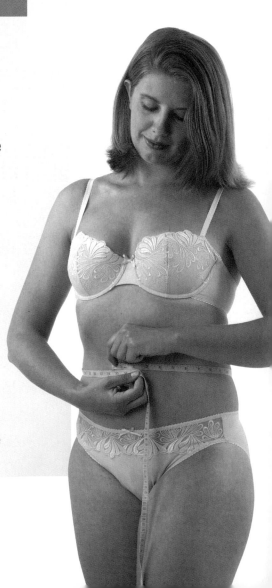

✓ Your weight-loss programme book or meeting may also advise you to take circumference measurements of upper arm and thighs. This can be an extra incentive, as these measurements in particular can give very pleasing results as the weeks progress!

**FACT**

Forget the old wives' tale of putting a finger behind the tape measure, tolerances are already built into garments. For instance, if your waist measures 32 inches, which makes you a fashion size 16, the actual waist measurement on the size 16 garment will be about 33.5 inches. If a generously styled, size 14 fashion blouse fits you, but you are a size 18, this isn't a garment you are 'getting away with'. This is a garment that is designed to be loose fitting and flowing, and will look awful stretched beyond recognition.

After your weekly measurement check, compare your measurements with a typical fashion sizing chart. All mail order catalogues carry them (near the back) and most stores have them but they're not often on view. Or ask in your favourite store and an assistant should be able to oblige you.

| Order size | | 6 | 8 | 10 | 12 | 14 | 16 | 18 | 20 | 22 | 24 | 26 | 28 | 30 | 32 |
|---|---|---|---|---|---|---|---|---|---|---|---|---|---|---|---|
| To fit bust | (cms) | 77 | 81 | 86 | 91 | 96 | 102 | 108 | 113 | 119 | 124 | 129 | 134 | 139 | 144 |
| | (ins) | 30¼ | 32 | 34 | 36 | 38 | 40 | 42½ | 44½ | 47 | 49 | 51 | 53 | 55 | 57 |
| To fit waist | (cms) | 57 | 61 | 66 | 71 | 76 | 81 | 89 | 94 | 102 | 107 | 112 | 117 | 122 | 127 |
| | (ins) | 22½ | 24 | 26 | 28 | 38 | 32 | 35 | 37 | 40 | 42 | 44 | 46 | 48 | 50 |
| To fit hips | (cms) | 82 | 86 | 91 | 96 | 101 | 107 | 113 | 118 | 124 | 129 | 134 | 139 | 144 | 149 |
| | (ins) | 32½ | 34 | 36 | 38 | 40 | 42 | 44½ | 46½ | 49 | 51 | 53 | 55 | 57 | 59 |

| choosing the right leg length | size | (XS) ex-short | (S) short | (R) regular | (L) long | (XL) ex-long |
|---|---|---|---|---|---|---|
| | inside leg | 25" | 27" | 29" | 31" | 33" |

A typical fashion sizing chart.

They may also know the company sizing policy and be able to give you specialist advice. (Don't forget, it's not unusual to find that you are a different size in clothes from different stores.) This will help you to keep track of when your clothes are becoming baggy and unflattering, so you can take action to make sure you stay stylish, looking and feeling great.

## Don't forget your bras!

It used to be a struggle to find pretty larger styles of bra, but not any more. There are many designer labels and celebrity brands these days; different effects for minimising or maximising; and a variety of fabrics, laces and embroideries. And it's amazing how much difference a properly-fitting bra can make to your appearance, your comfort and your confidence – and according to research, 70% of us are wearing the wrong size! Here's how to tell if your bra doesn't fit properly:

✓ When you stand side-on at a mirror, the strap around your body rides up at the back.

✓ Underwires dig in, rub or poke out at the front.

✓ Your breasts bulge over the top of the cups, creating a visible line under tops.

It can be quite difficult to measure yourself for a bra, so it's best to use a free bra-fitting service in a trusted department store, such as Marks &

Spencer. If you are big-boobed and feel self-conscious, you could go to a shop that specialises in large sizes, such as Evans or Bravissimo – they will have seen it all before. Once you've been measured and are happy with the fit, remember that that size may only be relevant and used again for a similar style of bra. A completely different bra style may require a size up or down.

It's amazing how much difference a properly-fitting bra can make to your appearance, your comfort and your confidence.

If you're determined to measure yourself, you could access an online fitting guide on the internet, such as the bra size calculator at www.figleaves.com/uk.
Alternatively, measure yourself as described overleaf, using a soft tape-measure:

Bra straps that dig in often mean a larger cup size is required rather than a size-up in band size.

✓ Measure around your chest under your breasts, at the level where the lowest part of your bra should sit. Try not to let the tape slip down at the back. Take the measurement in inches – if it's an even number, add four. If it's an odd number, add five. The resulting number is your band size – for instance, 36, 38, 40, 42 etc.

✓ Now measure around the fullest part of your breasts – you want a snug but not squashed fit. Take your band size away from this bust measurement. If the two are the same, you are an A cup. If your bust size is one inch larger than your band size, you are a B cup . . . two inches larger and you are a C cup . . . three inches larger and you are a D cup . . . four inches larger and you are a DD cup . . . five inches larger and you are an E cup . . . six inches larger and you are an F cup – and so on through the cup sizes.

Don't forget that you can be different sizes in bras from different stores, just as you can for other clothes. And your bra size will change dramatically as you lose weight, so re-measure yourself regularly. However, if you take time and trouble to make sure your bras are the right size, it can make a hugely visible difference to your overall look, starting right now.

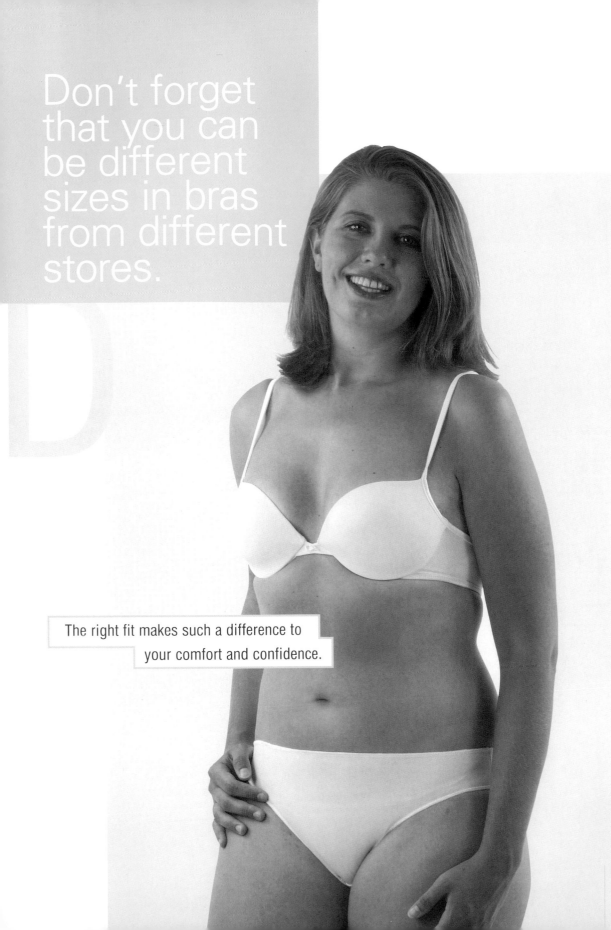

Don't forget that you can be different sizes in bras from different stores.

The right fit makes such a difference to your comfort and confidence.

## STEP 3 – Your lifestyle

Who are you? Where do you spend most of your time? To find out, divide up the time you spend on different aspects of your life. There are 168 hours in a week, and we spend up to 60 hours asleep – including the occasional lie-in, if we're lucky! Perhaps you spend 40 to 60 hours working and travelling? Maybe 10 hours socialising? Maybe 30 hours on essential chores and family concerns? Perhaps you have 8 hours of leisure time?

Now look at your wardrobe. With the information you have about how your life divides up, do the garments on the rail truly reflect what's going on? If your working life takes up half your working week, are half of the clothes and outfits in front of you dedicated to that purpose – or do your work outfits take up less space than your party gear? Are there things on the rail that have never been worn? Do you have a 'thin' section of clothes which you bought as incentives, to 'slim into'? Are there things on the rail that you just cannot bear to part with, because you've got an unnecessary emotional attachment to them? Own up! You know in your heart of hearts that if your wardrobe works for your lifestyle, it's going to help you look and feel better. If you look and feel better, you will perform better – at work, at home, with friends. Rebalancing the sections of your

> If your wardrobe works for your lifestyle, it's going to help you look and feel better.

wardrobe can give you a much more positive outlook on your life in general. It will also free up vital space for new outfits, which you never dreamed you'd be able to wear, to gradually take their rightful place there. So let's tackle it . . .

## STEP 4 — Your wardrobe

We're aiming for a happy-to-use wardrobe that's tailored to you. So its existing contents need to be assessed in detail before it can go through the transformation you yourself are going through. This process will help make the way ahead clearer. It may also often make the phrase (or excuse, if you're honest) 'I haven't got anything to wear' completely redundant.

Going through all your garments will take time, so give yourself a whole day off other duties to attend to it. Too indecisive? Enlist the help of a trusted friend — but be prepared to accept their judgement about what suits you.

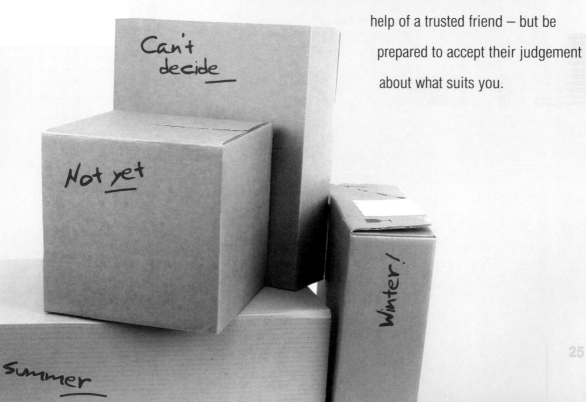

And don't take it too personally if she/he doesn't seem to like much of what you have – they are unselfishly giving up a whole day to help you! Bear in mind that this is not an easy task by any means; there may come a time mid-afternoon when you want to plonk yourself down amid the clothes and have a nap or a weep! But if you get really stuck in and concentrate on the job in hand, you'll get there in the end. Keep focussed on how uplifting it will feel when you've finished.

## Sort out your seasons

First things first . . . bring all your outfits out into the open from drawers, cupboards, rails, bin bags and boxes, etc., and put them on the floor, or the bed, or wherever. Now, start to divide everything into two seasons: spring/summer and autumn/winter. Keep out the current season's clothes, but fold or hang or bag (or send to the cleaners) the other season's clothes and put them in a space well out of reach, such as in the loft or under the bed. Don't keep them in your 'dressing area'; the temptation to keep dipping into them will be too great. We don't need to sort out what fits you, or doesn't fit you, in this discarded season's wardrobe; by the time you're ready to look at this lot again, you'll have changed

For this current season's clothes, divide your rail space into 'subject matter' sections which relate to your day-to-day life.

What to wear when you are losing weight
now

shape! Don't think twice – just do it. It's not as scary a procedure as actually throwing away, because you can come back to these clothes when the weather changes.

## Sort out your sections

For this current season's clothes, divide your rail space into 'subject matter' sections which relate to your day-to-day life. Work, casual, social, vegging out and maybe sport relate to most. Casual, social, red carpet and cruise may relate to some! But call each section whatever you like; you, and only you, know and can decide where that pilled, acrylic cardigan really belongs!

Don't throw anything away yet, but force yourself to stop and view each section with suspicion. For instance, there may be twelve pairs of baggy trackie bottoms which you just wear about the house, that you have always thought would be good enough for the gym – whenever you get around to joining! But think: are they really good enough for the gym? If we know deep down that what we are wearing is only a nano-second away from being destined for the cat basket, then we'll be disinclined to step out of our back door. The baggy trackie bottoms may be better replaced by 'intelligent'-fibre workout bottoms which cleverly wick away moisture and don't get wet if you build up a sweat. Clothing which helps you keep cool and stay attractive will encourage you to get out and exercise – whether it's to the gym or for a brisk walk around the block.

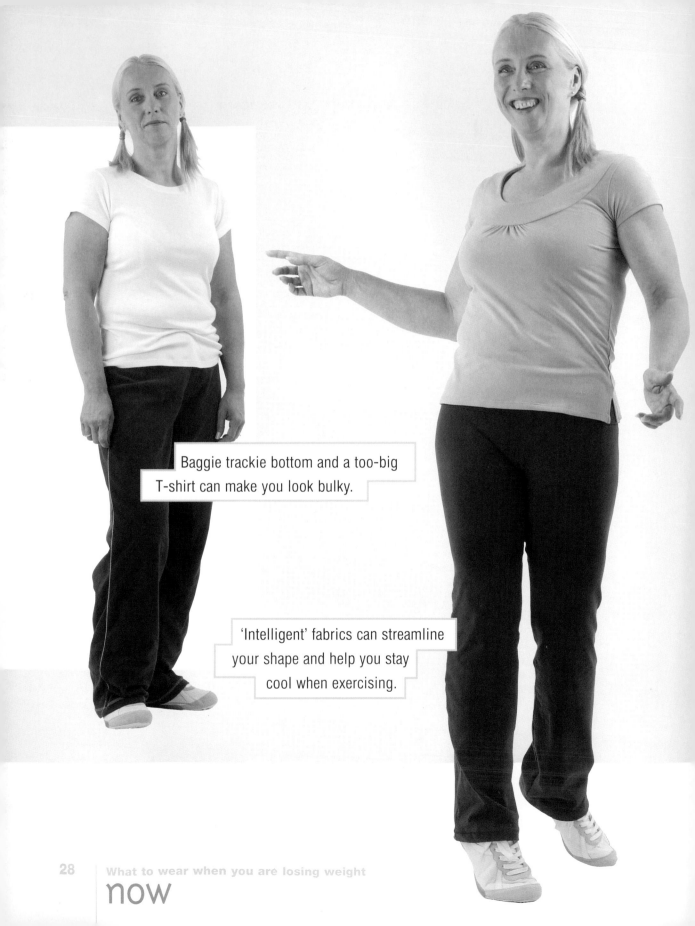

Baggie trackie bottom and a too-big T-shirt can make you look bulky.

'Intelligent' fabrics can streamline your shape and help you stay cool when exercising.

What to wear when you are losing weight
now

Ever wondered why there are so many sleeveless styles on offer in larger sizes when many of us want to cover up our wobbly arms? Garments with sleeves are one of the most returned garments in the fashion industry because of problems with the fit – our arms and shoulders are all different shapes and sizes, and even our posture can create problems with fit. Manufacturers don't want returns, they want to make money, so they often create larger-sized clothes without sleeves. Unfortunately, this is rarely flattering for us . . .

## What fits?

Now's the time to divide your wardrobe into what fits you now, what's too big and you're saving for the 'bad' days, and what's really too small if you're being honest. Bag up the too-small pieces in transparent garment bags, but keep them on your rail – it's a 'you can look but don't touch' incentive; when what's left on your rail becomes baggy, you have permission to open the bags and try these too-tight things on.

What you've got on your rails right now completely simplifies the getting-dressed procedure; all you have is this choice, however limited, so less time is wasted in making a decision. Treasure this time saved; it frees up minutes, which will amount to hours, which can be better spent on new enjoyable activities, such as pampering treats.

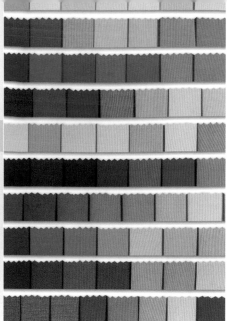

## Divide into colours

Divide each section of your wardrobe into similar colours. Within each colour, divide again into plain fabrics and patterns.

What are we left with? Ideally, your 'core' collection is comprised of classic colours and shapes which may last several years or more. It's even better if the garments interact with each other – this jacket works with its matching trousers, but also with the skirt from that suit, and the jersey trousers from that knit two-piece. This is what designers call a capsule wardrobe. A classic 'core' can be refreshed and revived each season by adding the latest accessories – tying a scarf an up-to-date way, or teaming an item with chunky jewellery or brightly coloured tights.

If what you're looking at right now is in bold print, has a strong weave or fancy texture, then these garments date way faster than the classics. Bought only a couple of seasons ago? You may get away with it. If it's any older, then what you're looking at is probably a dated shape as well as a dated cloth, even if you think it's a classic. It's time to now think about ditching these garments for good.

## Reject the rubbish

Now cast your eyes over each garment left on the rail for signs of pilling, drooping hems, missing buttons, indelible staining, rips and tears. Ask yourself if each problem is repairable, and, if so, is it worth taking the time to fix it yourself (or ask a friend), or spending the money on it at the 'repairs' section of the dry cleaner's. If it's not worth it, and you're an experienced sewer, the temptation will be strong to save anything about to be discarded to make into something else: a mat or a tablecloth. By all means do so, but know your own limitations. Will it lie around in the sewing basket for a number of years gathering more dust?

Now's the time to bag-up rejected garments. Take them to the charity shop if they're in good condition, or to the clothing bank at the recycling centre if not. It can be hard to throw away a garment when you remember how much you paid for it, but if you've got a lot of wear and some good times out of it, then it's earned its keep. If it's a desperately painful exercise, award yourself something that's up to date as a treat.

## Getting the balance right

The balance of garments which remain in your wardrobe is highly likely to be incorrect, now you're familiar with your actual requirements, but this 'core' is where all your key looks for the forthcoming season will spring from. This core wardrobe isn't going to be the wardrobe you'll travel with on your entire weight-loss journey, but it's a basis. This rail is going to see so many changes; think of it as a railway station. This is standing stock; other garments will visit for a short while; some will return as the seasons change; and some smaller-size things will be in temporary residence while you can make use of them. But, eventually, all the garments will leave the station, never to return!

**FACT**

The perfect core wardrobe for anyone, regardless of size, is a few best-you-can-afford, timeless pieces: a trouser suit (with skirt, if you've got good legs), three or four tops which can be worn with or without a jacket, three or four pairs of casual trousers, a couple of crisp white shirts, some knits and T-shirts and a smattering of day-into-evening styles.

This core wordrobe isn't going to be the wardrobe you'll travel with on your entire weight-loss journey, but it's a basis.

Take some time at the weekend to prepare your outfits for the week ahead. Then you'll be able to experiment with accessories, jewellery and different pairs of shoes and tights. Enjoy wearing your core clothes, however old they are, because you're like an artist-in-residence in them, temporarily existing in their space whilst you recreate yourself!

## STEP 5 — Your best bits

Everybody has a 'best bit'. Maybe it's your great legs? Twinkling eyes? Beautiful skin? Is your bosom worth showing off? Have you got a lovely smile? Does your hair make you resemble a goddess? Do you have an effusive personality?

Clothes shopping can be particularly hard if we've gained weight and feel at an especially low ebb. It can be tempting to 'disappear' in the crowd, and experience relief and pleasure at getting home – 'Ooh, I'm glad that's over'. However, if you focus on making the most of your best bits, it should help you to enjoy the outing itself. And recognising attributes and developing the skill of buying clothes to show them off is an important key to being and feeling stylish. The best thing about 'best bits' is that, even at this stage, when you perhaps feel you don't have any, they will be starting to emerge very soon!

**FACT**

Brunette, blonde, redhead, grey? Fair, olive, sallow, ruddy? Different colours work well or disastrously on us, because of our natural colouring and our build. We're often too easily persuaded into black because of its slimming effect. But colours can complement us too - it's just a matter of knowing which ones suit us. Try holding different colours to your face and check which look best against your complexion and eye colour. Try the scarf department of your nearest department store; it's the greatest abundance of colour, and no one knows you've no intention of buying!

## STEP 6 — Exercise

Exercise is vital in your new 'me' regime. As well as helping keep many diseases at bay, and making us more toned and flexible, it will reduce stress by releasing endorphins (the feel-good chemicals we all have in our bodies). Feeling good means we are more likely to stick to our weight-loss programme.

Walking is the easiest exercise to incorporate into your life. It's low-impact, so it doesn't cause any unnecessary strain on joints, provided it's done at a gentle pace to begin with. It's also vital to use supportive trainers or your most comfortable shoes. Just start by walking for 10 minutes a day. Begin slowly, to avoid cramp and stiffness, otherwise you'll be completely put off going out again tomorrow! Gradually work up to 15 minutes a day, then 20 minutes a day, until you manage a good 30 minutes a day or more. You may find it inspiring to arrange to walk with a friend. Devise a round-the-block route, with a few variants; if you pass by anything vaguely like a fish 'n' chip shop, kebab house, burger bar or Indian takeaway, take a deep breath and hurry on by. Buy a step counter and see how many steps you take on a typical walk. It will be a great encouragement to see that each week, you're beating the previous week's record.

# Walking is the easiest exercise to incorporate into your life.

Swimming is a low-impact aerobic exercise, meaning that it doesn't stress the joints or the spine, and it's a great workout for our heart and lungs. The water supports our bodies, whatever our size, so swimming is a great equaliser. Even if we can't swim, we can participate in aqua-aerobics classes, keeping our feet on the bottom of the pool. The resistance of the water as we move is like working with weights, so we'll develop a firmer and leaner frame. Water also allows us more movement than on land so our muscles can stretch and we'll increase our flexibility. All in all, the perfect exercise.

## STEP 7 — Grooming

Carrying extra weight can have a negative knock-on effect: we might feel we are unworthy of pampering, or we feel 'who's going to notice?' Not everyone falls prey to these feelings, but many do, and it's a hard hole to climb out of, if you're stuck deep down. Starting to look after your external body in the same way you are looking after your internal body with diet can have startlingly positive physical and mental changes.

> A new 'face' and new haircut creates the best possible diversionary tactic away from the body that's undergoing a change.

## Pamper yourself

There are days, we all have them, when it's a slopping about, no make-up, bad hair day, sure – but if there's even the slightest chance of being seen by anyone other than your very nearest and dearest, it's a positive step to make yourself look the best you can. There will have been times where you've wanted to hide away, but this 'now' time is a way of turning your back on the shrinking violet you sometimes want to be.

The makeover TV programmes wait until the last minute to reveal the hair and make-up changes, don't they? It causes the greatest whoops of delight because it's the most noticeable thing. Where do people look when they're talking to you? Your face, of course? A new 'face' and new haircut creates the best possible diversionary tactic away from the body that's undergoing a change. It's also the first physical change that you can make to show that a new you is on the way.

'Cleanse, cleanse again, tone and moisturise' are the skincare basics we all know about, but work in a deep facial cleanse once a week, too. Add a hair treatment, together with a weekly pedicure/manicure/depilatory session, and relaxing 'me' time into your schedule.

## The benefits of massage

As the inches drop off, if you've never had a massage then now is the time to book one. A massage is a great relaxation technique, especially if it becomes part of your regular feel-good rituals.

We all fight shy of taking our clothes off when we're not figure perfect, and to have a stranger not only look at us, but also touch our naked flesh and pummel all the wobbly bits, always seems way off limits at first. But the benefits of massage far outweigh any stress – which is in our minds after all.

Massage can vary from light brushstrokes on the skin to pressure into deep tissue, and the different strokes are designed to act on the muscular, nervous, circulatory and lymphatic systems. Opt for an independent therapist rather than a beauty salon treatment as your new therapist will be practised in a more holistic approach – the real meaning of therapy – and will begin to 'read' your body and

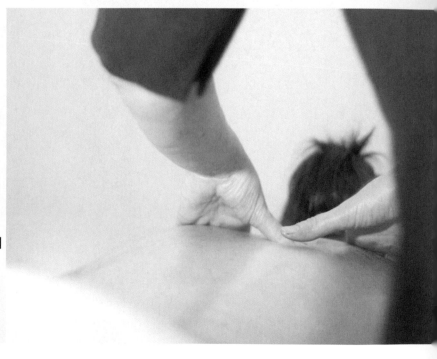

Make-up can disguise
how tired and washed
out we feel ... it can
help us look at the
world straight on.

concentrate on areas which are troublesome. As many massages include
the head and use oils, be prepared to leave with a Ken Dodd-type hairstyle.
Try to plan an appointment for later in the day, go straight home and have
an early night – a deep, sweet sleep is almost guaranteed. Drink water, too,
immediately afterwards to replace what you've lost. Do without and you
may suffer a slight headache.

## Make-up

Not wearing make-up can be a political stance, if you're so inclined; but
make-up is not our enemy – it's a very good ally. Make-up can disguise
how tired and washed out we feel; it can make us look alert, a lot prettier; it
can help us look at the world straight on.

We all look better with a bit of make-up, although there's a fine line between too much or too little. If you feel happy with your current look, fine; if not, take advantage of the makeover offers at most make-up counters in every department store. You don't feel as 'exposed' as you might think. There's also valuable advice to be gained by asking constant questions about how and why this or that product is used and how it's being applied. You'll learn more about your skin type and natural colouring, and what shades flatter, than any amount of experimentation at home – without the risk of having purchased an unsuitable product. Some product brands charge for the service; other brands provide it free, as long as you make a purchase. Think of it as an investment.

## Hair

It would be a shame to waste the air of experimentation about you now. So, however close you are to your existing hairdresser, and however much you feel disloyal by contemplating going anywhere else, now's the time to take advantage of the free consultation that most salons offer. You have no obligation, and all you're losing is your time. It gives you the power to make a really positive step; to change something that's perhaps become predictable, and to be adventurous. A trendy hairstyle disguises a not-so up-to-the-minute outfit. It can take years off your face and give you an instant style.

Draw an oval, an oblong, a circle, a square, a heart and a pear shape on a sheet of paper. These are the six most common face shapes. Draw the outlines of hairstyles on each and you'll see which style works best on each shape. The round face suits layers and a graduated cut to 'break up' the roundness. The square needs a side parting and a bit of curl to soften the very straight hairline and jawline. The heart-shape needs a centre parting and a chin-length style to add fullness and to even things out. The pear-shape needs a short style to balance a prominent jaw. The oval-shape suits almost any style, as well as scraped back.

Hairdressers are only human; a new hairdresser knows nothing about you initially. You can help by explaining your requirements as fully as you can, and by taking along pictures of styles you like. Try to take as bold a step as you dare! 'NOW' is starting to become 'THEN'!

# Success stories

**Name:** Aileen King
**Start weight:** 14 stone 13 pounds
**Weight now:** 10 stone 3 pounds
**Clothes size before:** 22
**Clothes size now:** 10 to 12
**Meeting:** Thundersley, Essex

I always struggled with my weight, and was known as 'the little big one' among family and friends. I was a 'secret eater' – if no one saw me eat junk food, takeaways, biscuits, crisps and chocolate, then I hadn't eaten it! Over the years, I tried numerous faddy diets, losing and regaining the weight I had lost – and then some!

Being diagnosed with breast cancer in October 2003 was a turning point. After surgery, chemotherapy and radiotherapy, I started to get strong and well; I was determined to survive. But I made up my mind that, having had one health scare, my weight was not going to cause others. I tried various unsupported diets and managed to lose a stone and a half, but then I got stuck – and decided to join Weight Watchers.

The Full Choice plan suited me best as no food was banned. After just Week Two I got my first Silver Seven – I felt very proud. I looked at every two-pound loss as another bag of sugar, and kept myself going by planning healthy meals and removing unhealthy temptations from my surroundings. I also created an 'emergency kit' at work of healthy snacks and meals held in store for busy days. As the weight came off, my skills with the sewing machine improved, and I enjoyed altering my clothes to my new shape. With my new-found confidence and the support of my husband and family, I started regular exercise at my local gym. The Weight Watchers meetings gave me the support and motivation I needed to put 'bad days' behind me and keep going.

Now friends I haven't seen for a long time can hardly recognise me – but I feel that I have got both myself and my life back.

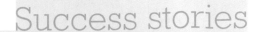

**Name:**             Helen Lane
**Start weight:**      12 stone 12 1/2 pounds
**Weight now:**        9 stone 11 pounds
**Clothes size before:**  16 to 18
**Clothes size now:**    10
**Meeting:**         Waltham Abbey, Essex

I had a clear reason for wanting to lose two stone – I wanted to lose my excess weight before having another baby. But I could not have done it without Weight Watchers. I loved the way the diet fitted me. I didn't have to eat anything I didn't like, and I didn't have to cook separate food for my family. The tips and motivation I gained from the meetings kept me going – and I enjoyed the social aspect too.

Once my baby was born, I returned to meetings after my six-week check to lose the 'baby weight'. My leader provided me with invaluable help as, like me, she is a mother of two. She has maintained her goal weight for more than seven years, so she speaks from personal experience and is a fantastic inspiration. She's helped me to lose three stone: two before I fell pregnant, and a stone afterwards.

Weight Watchers has become a way of life for me. The healthy eating and exercise plan is so easy to follow that I can enjoy special events such as holidays and birthdays without worrying about the pounds creeping on. The support I receive from meetings gives me the confidence and incentive to keep on track.

# Success stories

**Name:** Tina Gregory
**Start weight:** 13 stone 6½ pounds
**Weight now:** 11 stone 3 pounds
**Clothes size before:** 18 to 20
**Clothes size now:** 14
**Meeting:** Canvey Island, Essex

I joined Weight Watchers after seeing a photo of myself at my youngest son's christening. The pounds had piled on over a few years, but I had never really taken much notice. I was always too busy rushing around after my two little boys – I had thought that the 'baby weight' would disappear on its own. When I saw the christening photo, I couldn't believe what I was looking at. I realised that I had to take action – losing the weight was not just going to happen, and certainly no one was going to do it for me.

Like many people, I had lost weight with Weight Watchers before. And like many people, once I stopped attending meetings and paying attention to my food and exercise, the weight crept back on. But I wanted this time to be different. I wanted to lose all the weight I had to lose, once and for all – to reveal the shapely me I knew was lurking under there somewhere.

It took me a long year to reach my goal weight. I had good and not-so-good weeks, but following the Weight Watchers plan I was able to still live life to the full – and I got there in the end. As I lost the excess pounds I really gained confidence, and I actually began to enjoy buying clothes! Finally, I was asked to become a Weight Watchers leader. At first I couldn't imagine being an inspiration for others to lose weight, but here I am, two and a half years later, running five successful meetings a week.

# Recipes for success

Here are some favourite Weightwatcher recipes — simple and delicious.

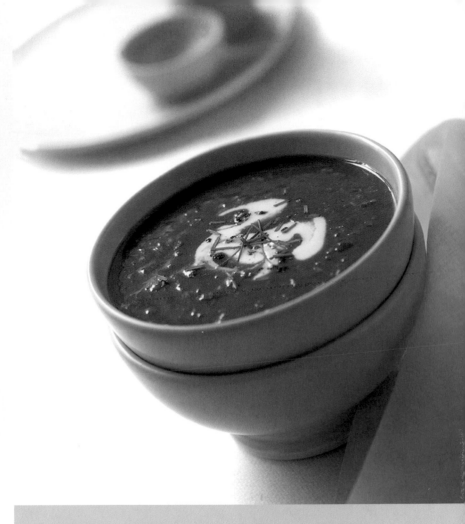

## Super speedy tomato soup

600 ml (1 pint) tomato juice

1/2 vegetable stock cube, dissolved in 4 tablespoons hot water

1 teaspoon garlic purée

1 teaspoon Tabasco sauce

1 tablespoon chopped fresh chives, basil or coriander

salt and freshly ground black pepper

2 tablespoons low-fat plain yogurt, to garnish

 serves 2  1 POINTS VALUE  Per serving  60 cals  V

- Preparation and cooking time 10 minutes.
- Freezing recommended.
- 1 1/2 *POINTS* values per recipe

This is the quickest home-made soup ever! It makes a very tasty light meal, snack or starter.

1   Put the tomato juice and stock into a saucepan and add the garlic purée and Tabasco sauce. Bring up to the boil, reduce the heat, then add most of the chopped chives, basil or coriander, reserving some for garnish.

2   Season the soup with salt and pepper, adding a few more drops of Tabasco sauce, if you like your food to be spicy.

3   Serve the soup, topping each portion with a tablespoon of yogurt, chopped fresh herbs and a little extra ground black pepper.

**Variation:** Instead of tomato juice, use V8 vegetable juice.

# Chilli beef burgers

1 small onion, diced

1 tablespoon Worcestershire
   sauce

350 g (12 oz) extra lean minced
   beef

1 pickled gherkin, chopped finely

1 teaspoon chilli flakes

1 egg, beaten

a few lettuce leaves, to garnish

serves 4 · 3½ POINTS VALUE · Per serving · 185 cals

- Preparation time 10 minutes.
- Cooking time 15 minutes.
- Freezing recommended.
- 14 **POINTS** values per recipe

Serve hot in a split bap with a few lettuce leaves, adding the **POINTS** as necessary.

1   Place the onion in a small pan with 2 tablespoons water and the Worcestershire sauce. Cover and cook gently for 2 to 3 minutes until softened. Drain and place in a mixing bowl.

2   Add the minced beef, gherkin, chilli flakes and egg. Mix well.

3   Divide the mixture into four even-sized burgers and grill under a medium heat for 5 minutes per side.

**Cook's note**: You could use lamb or turkey mince if preferred. The **POINTS** values per serving will be 4 with lamb and 2 1/2 with turkey. Flavour the lamb burgers with dried mint instead of chilli flakes and the turkey with wholegrain mustard.

# Broad bean and mint risotto

1 tablespoon olive oil

4 shallots, thinly sliced

1 garlic clove, peeled and crushed

225 g (8 oz) risotto rice

30 ml (1 fl oz) vermouth (optional)

700 ml (1 1/4 pints) vegetable stock

350 g (12 oz) broad beans, shelled

25 g (1 oz) fresh Parmesan, grated

2 tablespoons chopped fresh mint

serves 4 · 5½ POINTS VALUE · Per serving · 315 cals · V

- Preparation time 15 minutes
- Cooking time 30 minutes.
- Freezing recommended.
- 21 1/2 **POINTS** values per recipe

Shelling the broad beans is time-consuming but the end result with the bright green beans makes it really worthwhile. To save time, you could use frozen peas instead, but it won't be the same.

1   Heat the olive oil in a large pan and cook the shallots and garlic for 2 to 3 minutes, until just beginning to soften. Add the rice and stir well. Cook for a further 2 to 3 minutes.

2   Stir in the vermouth, if using. Then gradually add the stock a little at a time, waiting for what you add to be absorbed by the rice before adding more.

3   As you are adding the last of the stock, toss in the beans, Parmesan and mint. Continue cooking until the rice is creamy and tender. A successful risotto should also be a bit sloppy. It should take about 20 minutes in all.  Serve at once.

**Cook's note:** If you're freezing this, you may want to add some extra stock as you heat it through.

# Kidney bean and chilli pâté

1 teaspoon sunflower oil

1 small onion, chopped

1 garlic clove, crushed

1 teaspoon chilli flakes

425 g (15 oz) canned kidney beans, drained

125 g (4 1/2 oz) low-fat soft cheese

2 tablespoons freshly squeezed lemon juice

salt and freshly ground black pepper

serves 4 · 2 1/2 POINTS VALUE · Per serving · 120 cals · V

• Preparation time 10 minutes.

• Freezing recommended.

• 10 1/2 *POINTS* values per recipe

Spread on toast for a tasty starter or serve as a dip with a selection of veggies.

1   Heat the sunflower oil in a small pan and cook the onion, garlic and chilli flakes over a low heat for 5 minutes, until softened not browned.

2   Remove from the heat. Allow to cool a little, then transfer to a food processor with the drained kidney beans, low-fat soft cheese and lemon juice. Blend until smooth and season to taste.

3   Transfer to a serving dish and chill until ready to eat.

**Variation:** Other canned beans and spices can be substituted for the kidney beans and chilli, such as chick peas with ground coriander, or butter beans and cumin.

# Tiny cheesecake tarts

150 g (5 1/2 oz) sweet shortcrust pastry, thawed if frozen

100 g (3 1/2 oz) cottage cheese

1 small egg, beaten

25 g (1 oz) currants

25 g (1 oz) golden caster sugar

finely grated zest of 1 lemon

pinch of ground nutmeg

makes 12 · 2 POINTS VALUE · Per serving · 85 cals · V

• Preparation time 20 minutes.

• Cooking time 20–25 minutes.

• Freezing recommended.

• 21 1/2 *POINTS* values per recipe

Good for an Easter treat.

1   Preheat the oven to Gas Mark 4/180°C/350°F.

2   Roll out the pastry on a lightly floured surface. Use to line 12 small tartlet tins or a 12-hole patty tin, using a fork to prick the base of each one. Place the tins on a baking sheet.

3   Mix together the cottage cheese, egg, currants and sugar. Spoon the mixture into the pastry-lined patty tins. Sprinkle each one with lemon zest and ground nutmeg.

4   Bake for 20–25 minutes, until set and golden brown. Serve warm or cold.

sometime soon

ometime soon som

**Part 2**

# Simple alterations

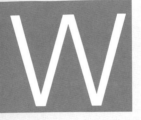hat's left of your wardrobe after the great sort-out of the section may not seem much, but at least it's a more uncluttered and efficient use of space. It's time-saving too: you know what's there fits and, thanks to your efforts, fits better than before. The items that have previously been tight are now a joy to wear – the single-breasted jacket that used to only fasten at the top now fastens on the bottom button too; the skirt that you could zip three-quarters of the way now skims the hips, and you can not only fasten the clip, but there's room to spare.

It's at this stage that it's tempting to throw a couple of items away – but don't, not just yet. The trick now is to separate garments with worthwhile fabric or styles that haven't dated into an 'altering' pile.

## Altering baggy bottoms

Where are you losing the weight from first? Is it the derrière where you've first noticed a difference? When it comes to trousers and skirts, what's baggy whilst you're standing up but a bit tight when you're sitting down will last a while longer. However, if you can pinch spare fabric both standing and sitting, then some simple sewing alterations will give your favourite bottoms a little more longevity. Remember, what you can alter

## sometime soon

now, saves buying too much in this interim stage and stores up any potential spending for when you really need a shopping boost.

Here's the best way to tackle a baggy trousers and skirts. Turn the trousers or skirt inside out and put them on, taking care to fasten them normally. If you're an experienced seamstress, you may decide to remove the waistband, take a few inches off either side, and re-set it. As with all sewing jobs, make sure that you choose matching threads, so repairs and alterations are less obvious. If you're a less-experienced sewer, you have two options. The first option is to leave the waistband as it is, but wear a belt over it. Longer-length belts are easily bought from plus-size specialist stores, or you could try a man's belt. Remember, this is a transitory use item, and if you cover your waist and tum with a long top, no one will see it. The second option is to simply chop through the waistband taking some off either side. But this option will only suit hand-sewers – the resulting bunch may not actually fit under a sewing machine 'foot', and even if it does, the brute strength needed to go through four layers of fabric plus interfacing may harm the machine.

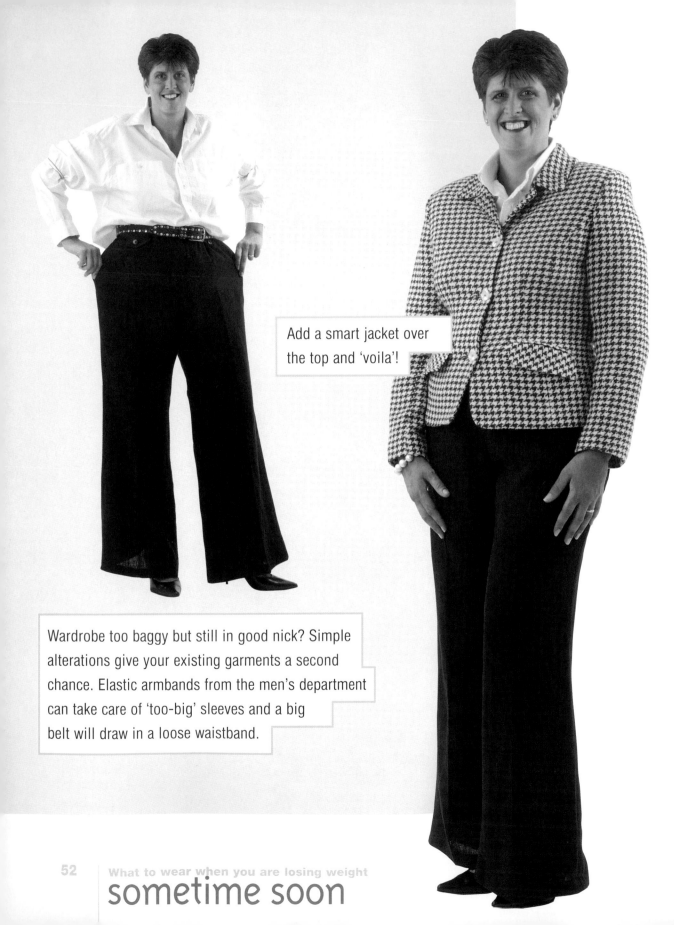

Add a smart jacket over the top and 'voila'!

Wardrobe too baggy but still in good nick? Simple alterations give your existing garments a second chance. Elastic armbands from the men's department can take care of 'too-big' sleeves and a big belt will draw in a loose waistband.

What to wear when you are losing weight
# sometime soon

Congratulations if you have got elasticised-waistband styles. All you need to do here is unpick the central seam, grab the elastic, snip a few inches off and sew it back up. If you're in a hurry and the elastic is thin enough, you could even tie it, pop it back into the opening and sew up the seam.

When it comes to baggy skirts, it's fairly simple to pin the amount of side seam to be taken in, then sew along it. But you'll notice that trouser-legs are an unusual construction on most styles: the front half is smaller than the back. So in order to keep the taking-in of side seams as even as possible, start to pin excess fabric equally on both outside and inside leg seams, front and back legs. If not done evenly, the legs will 'twist' which makes them unsightly and uncomfortable. Test the 'give' as you go along, making sure you're able to sit. (Squat! No one's watching!) Stop the taking-in by the knee in a graduated fluid line; this won't spoil the overall look.

## Altering baggy tops

Are you losing off your shoulders and bosom? If so, garments will suddenly develop longer arm lengths; what's been stretched, suddenly hangs. Simple sleeves will just require a hem, either machined or hand-sewn. Cuffs are more troublesome, but like we used a belt to make an instant improvement, what about elastic armbands from the men's department? These can be an instant stylish touch.

Taking-in favourite jersey and T-shirt tops is best done on a sewing machine using an 'elastic-give' stitch and a special rounded-end jersey needle to prevent tearing and laddering the fabric (jersey is knitted using the same techniques and fibres as tights and stockings). So turn the garment inside out and put it on and, preferably with the help of a pal, start to pin excess fabric in an even line all the way along the side seams and underarms, and make a note of how much to take up and hem the sleeve length.

## Call in the professionals

Of course, there are garments such as tailored jackets and winter coats that are just too complicated in structure and detail to make any sort of alterations without professional help. This is where alteration-tailors and private dressmakers and the seamstresses attached to many dry-cleaning firms become useful. It can seem like an expensive procedure, but weigh it up. In comparison to buying a completely new garment, and especially if the fabric is good quality and in good condition, professional help may be worth considering. If the alteration will cost more than to buy new, then put that money aside for a replacement!

A tip for home-sewers: editor of *Sew Today*, Julie Watkins, says 'You should never choose a pattern based on what you would buy from retailers, as they vary. Take your own body measurements and compare them to the appropriate sizes on the measurement charts found in each of the pattern catalogues, Butterick, McCalls and Vogue Patterns'.

## To shop or not to shop

What are we left with now in your wardrobe? A smaller rail of wearables for the moment, hopefully. Ask yourself some serious questions. Does this fulfil your requirements for your typical week? Office-bound? Are there at least four passable outfits (three for wearing during the week, with one in the laundry or at the dry cleaner's?) Are there a couple of dressier pieces for a bit of a social life? Three or four casual outfits for the weekend? Is there something that you're really lacking, or can you hold off spending money at the shops for the time being? Think of the pros and cons of holding off any purchases . . .

Still at the in-between stage, but wanting a fashion boost? Robe, kimono, wrap and apron-style tops and knits can all be bought in a smaller size than you are right now to give your wardrobe a bit more of a seasonal or colour boost; just don't fasten them! They're going to fit perfectly soon and if they get too big they'll still be a valid piece for your wardrobe – just wear them over a lambswool or cashmere or angora roll neck in winter, or layer them over vests and tops in summer to use them as a summer coat.

Pros:

✓ Not buying something now means you'll have more money to spend at a later, 'slimmer' date.

✓ Your body shape is changing. If you buy something now, it won't fit soon, and then it will have been a waste of money.

## Cons:

✗ Your wardrobe has taken something of a battering and basically you're bored with it. Seeing something new hanging up will cheer you up no end.

✗ You've thrown away the top of one outfit and the bottom of another . . . A couple of tops which co-ordinate with both could bring the separate pieces together and – voila – whole new outfits!

There's no right answer! You make your own decision!

# sometime soon

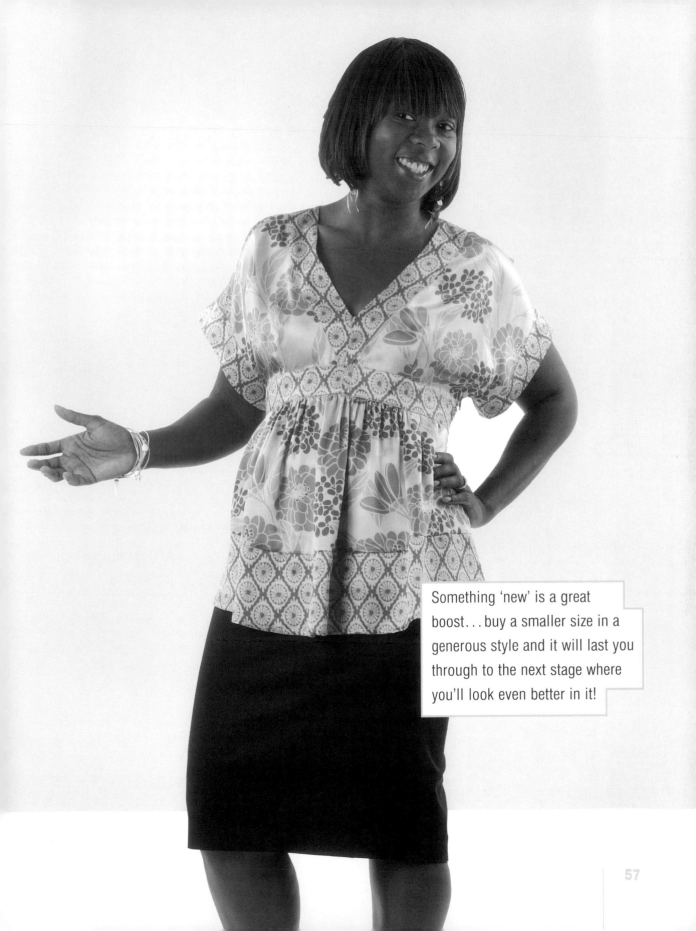

Something 'new' is a great boost... buy a smaller size in a generous style and it will last you through to the next stage where you'll look even better in it!

57

## Who's looking even better by the minute?

We all lose weight from different areas at first, and even one body may not change in all areas all at the same time. The bum may stubbornly sit whilst all around slims down. The shoulder blades may suddenly appear, but it's too early to reveal them in a strappy top. Take a considered, thoughtful approach to when you are ready to expose body parts that haven't been exposed before – your décolleté? Your arms? Your waist? Your ankles? Don't be impatient, you can reveal the new you little by little. Even if you don't feel ready to reveal your knees or bare your arms, you can show off your improved overall shape with a new closer-fitting garment. Others will see that you're losing weight by the way your face looks and how well your clothes fit. Imagine their surprise!

> Don't be impatient, you can reveal the new you little by little.

## Hitting the high street

Like it or not, we are an ever-increasingly consumer society and clothing is abundant, full of 'must-haves' and the season's 'best-buys'. As the pounds disappear, we could shop till we drop! The good news is that most high-street brands are beginning to recognise that the average UK female is size 16, 5' 4" high and a D cup. They are beginning to add size 18 and even 20

What to wear when you are losing weight
## sometime soon

into their fashion ranges. However, there's a cautionary note. Many brands design in sample sizes, an 8 or a 10. These designs often tend to lose a little of their cuteness and delicacy as the sizes creep up. So it's important to be able to judge a garment on its merits, rather than just to pounce on it because it's got the right size label. Ask yourself: does it actually do anything for you? And will it add any 'value' (not monetary, but in terms of usage) to your existing garments? Be ruthless about clothing; if it's not perfect for you, don't buy it just for the sake of buying something.

## 'In-between stage' shopping tips

It's currently in vogue to have a mix of high fashion, high street, interchangeable basics and supermarket affordables, together with a bit of designer if we're lucky and a little bit of vintage. Of course, we all have different tastes and varying budgets. We all put things together in different ways. However, there are a few style tips that can help us make the most of ourselves, regardless of our personal preferences and spending ability. The main trick is to aim to balance your body by creating an equal proportion between your top and bottom half. If your top half is smaller than the bottom (a typical pear-shape), then lighter, brighter colours worn on top and darks on the bottom will create balance. If you are top-heavy, the opposite will work for you.

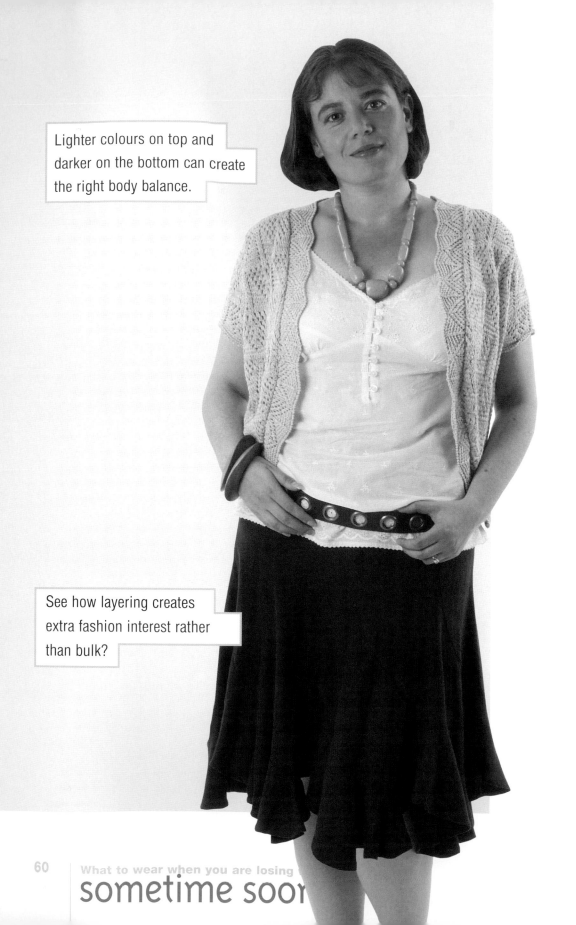

Lighter colours on top and darker on the bottom can create the right body balance.

See how layering creates extra fashion interest rather than bulk?

sometime soor

## Silhouette-skimming, figure-flattering

Always be wary of tight-fitting clothes until you've reached your goal weight. We can fool ourselves that close-fitting stretch garments are flattering because to a certain extent they hold us in. However, if you are carrying extra weight, there is the danger that tight becomes taut – stretch garments can easily look stretched beyond their capability! Instead, look for fabrics that skim the body – like fine knits and silks. Such garments will hint at your changing shape. They are particularly useful when you're losing your 'love handles' and that extra on your upper arms. If you previously wore clothes like these covered with a jacket on top, try wearing them on their own, unhidden. This will herald a major shift in your journey.

Also experiment with layering. Try to create interesting layers, say a square-cut vest top under a deep-V, fine wool, slightly shaped sweater or under a loose, kimono wide-sleeve top. This would look less bulky than a single layer tent-shape, plus it would have more visual interest and appear as if more thought had gone into the look. It's time to change from being an 'I just threw it on' type to an 'I chose this specially' type.

## 'In-between' tops

Continue to look for tops that cover your bottom; but too long – such as calf-length – and you'll look shorter. Overshirts and kaftan-shapes work well around the hips. Tunics, coat-dresses and safari styles all work well just at knee-length with trousers. An empire-line which fits neatly under the bust keeps the attention on the upper part of the body, shows off the bosom and disguises a non-existent waistline.

Crop cardigans have a similar effect and also help disguise less-than-perfect arms.

Delicate strap tops belong on others for the moment; there's a danger of looking strained and precarious rather than 'pretty' at this stage – but your time will soon come! At this stage in our journey, long sleeves are far more slimming than short. Even the slimmest, turn-back cuff adds length to the arm. Bell and long, fluted sleeves also help balance a heavier upper arm, but, boy, are they irritating to the more practical (they do have a habit of trailing in your dinner!). Instead, you could try a rolled-up sleeve worn with a long T-shirt underneath and a couple of chunky bangles; what you're doing is creating interest at the wrist and diverting attention from the top.

When it comes to necklines, lower necklines generally help break up the top half of the body and take attention away from the tum. Deep Vs, scoop necks, sweethearts and cowls are all flattering to a larger frame. Be wary of crew necks; worn on their own, they can create a boxy effect and make you look very 'square', especially if you have a large bosom. However, teamed with an additional softer garment with a deep V-shape (say a waistcoat, another piece of knitwear or an overshirt) they can look dramatic. Want a

sometime soon

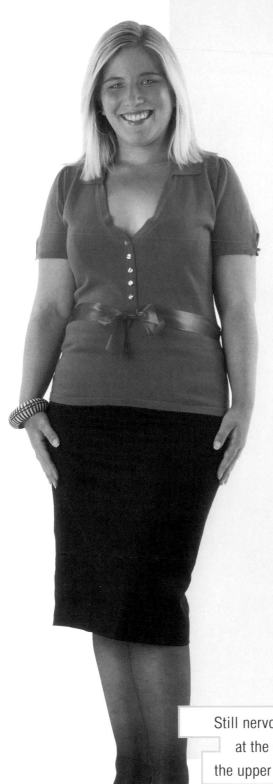

higher collar? Nehru or oriental collars are more flattering in general than crew necks, and much more interesting. Left unbuttoned, they create a deep long line with the same visual effect as the V.

## 'In-between' bottoms

If your waist doesn't diminish as quickly as you thought, low-waisted jeans and trousers might be a bit of a godsend. But wear a top long enough to cover the divide; never ever reveal what's going on underneath! To add length and slimness to the whole leg, avoid Capri-length styles; try long-leg straight styles or wide-leg styles almost skimming the ground. These add length and slimness to the whole leg and make the bottom look flatter. If you are tall, you could also try a trendy wide turn-up jean which draws the eye downward rather than looking full-on at the wider thigh.

If your pins are worthy of seeing, then do wear a skirt – if you're still a bit shy, try 60-denier tights.

Still nervous about legs? A lower neckline, a visual feature at the waist and a below-the-knee style concentrates the eye on the upper rather than lower body.

The most flattering length is often just below the knee. Calf-length straight styles teamed with knee-length boots are a stylish alternative to trousers and do a great job at disguising less-than-slim legs; but beware of slits in the back and sides, if you don't want others to glimpse a leg that's not ready just yet to be revealed to the world. To play safe, choose an A-line shape. Don't be afraid of a little embellishment or embroidery on the hem to make it less boring; this is also another good trick which helps draw the eye down to the bottom of the skirt, rather than resting on the fullest part of the figure, the hips.

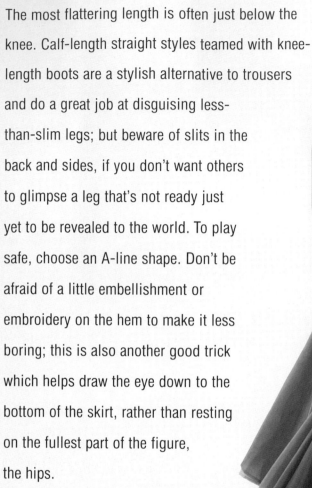

A-line skirts and fine layers move seductively and are very flattering.

What to wear when you are losing weight
## sometime soon

## Need help?

You've probably heard about personal shoppers and thought, 'Oh, I'll never get a look in . . . there must be a waiting list . . . they couldn't help me . . .' Well, you could be wrong! Personal shoppers are tireless, intensively trained individuals in most department stores who offer a mostly free service designed to help you put together an outfit that's right for you. It's usually a no-obligation-to-buy service, so what's to lose? As there's no obligation to buy, there's also certainly no obligation to take on board the advice you're given, but you may be taken by surprise at how astute these people can be.

Surely it would be interesting to hear what a stranger might suggest for your new look? It's a totally honest, unbiased viewpoint, rather than biased comments from friends and family (although given with the best intentions). You might even find the process fun!

Most department stores offer personal shopping as an appointment service rather than a 'drop in' facility. Choose a store according to your dress size at this stage; there are many stores that cater for up to size 22. Don't choose a store that isn't to your taste. There'll be nothing there for you, however well it fits. Try to time your visit to a personal shopper after a recent hairdo and with full make-up, looking your very best. Expect to be treated like a VIP, with a one-to-one consultation, a private changing area, refreshments, and the satisfaction of knowing that someone else is running round the store choosing on your behalf. Go with it, and enjoy the experience.

# Grooming

You've been eating more healthily for a while now, and it must be beginning to show through a clearer complexion and brighter eyes. You'll have more energy, too, with all that dietary goodness coursing through your veins. It's time to take advantage once more of what's happening to our hair, skin and nails.

## Reassess your hair

If you took the advice from the earlier section to try a new hairdresser, then it's time to make a return visit – or try somewhere new once more, for a fresh opinion. Take some pictures of styles you like cut-out from magazine

sometime soon

# As we're losing weight, our cheekbones are appearing, our jaws are becoming more angular and our features are becoming more defined.

pages, as a starting point to talk about – but leave yourself open to advice. This is perhaps scary, but can also be an exhilarating experience. Paying more for a creative director than a less experienced stylist could be a good investment. And be prepared to throw your carefully collected pictures and well-rehearsed words out of the window at an award-winning, reputable salon where there is a stylist you trust – he or she will, quite rightly, feel that they can judge the style best for you.

As we're losing weight, our cheekbones are appearing, our jaws are becoming more angular and our features are becoming more defined. But perhaps our faces are still a little rounder than we would like? The hairstyle we need now is one that creates length instead of width, to slim the face. An obvious no-no is a big and bubbly style, adding roundness to roundness. A good hairdresser will try to give extra height on the crown, keep length at the nape of the neck, and take excess width off the sides – often with the sides tucked behind the ears or cut short around the ears. (This maximises the effect of earrings too.) Avoid styles where the hair falls on to the cheeks, unless it's a wispy, delicate touch on a shorter style which makes the whole look much more feminine. Asymmetrical styles are also good for round faces as they counteract the roundness with their imbalance.

Remember, you can make your chosen or recommended hairstyle as interesting as you like by using products to create texture and also experimenting with colour – highlights or lowlights, choppy or block, whatever the latest style is. If you have permanent colour applied, be prepared (financially as well as time-wise) for maintenance treatments every six weeks. Roots start to be noticeable after three weeks or so and although touch-ups can be done at home, an overall colour will have to be re-done at intermittent intervals due to the effects of regular shampooing plus the fading effects of the sun. The important thing is that you're beginning to like changes and become excited by being adventurous. It's a good step to take.

## Keep busy with beautifying routines

Perhaps none of us can fit in a beautifying routine every day, but do try to fit in two or three sessions a week of dedicated pamper time. It keeps hands and thoughts busy away from snacking and, as more improvements occur, the less inclined we'll be to spoil our progress.

Reward your results so far by buying a robe – a new dressing gown,

# Start thinking of yourself as a priority rather than the last one on the list.

kimono, a kaftan or even a retro hostess gown! We're not talking nightie or jim-jams; this garment is to visually signify the change from daytime duty-time to me-pampering time, to alert your family, partner, flatmates or pets, and to put you in the mood to concentrate on yourself. There are always jobs to do . . . but start thinking of yourself as a priority rather than the last one on the list. What you're doing doesn't happen without a lot of effort. And the more effort made, the quicker and clearer the result.

The gown on, the hairband intact; you're ready for an improvement session — and it's up to you what you choose. Should you concentrate on nails tonight? Or a pedicure? A facial perhaps? A deep-conditioning treatment for the hair? Or what about a complete home spa evening? There're plenty of kits around — some complete with their own aromatherapy candle — and all devoid of calorific temptations . . .

## A manicure isn't just for nails

If you wear rings, you'll notice that they're beginning to be no longer tight — you're able to turn them to the point of beginning to slip off. This is another little feel-good boost, but what of your hands in general? Hands hold a secret — they give away our true age! A bit of little-and-often manicure care will go some way to maintaining our new well-groomed image. For a little bit of hand luxury, you could massage in nightly a rich handcream, then wear cotton gloves overnight. For nails, try a regular massage of cuticle cream or oil and a weekly push-back using a rubber-tipped cuticle stick. To tackle nail discolouration, try a specialist whitener or a small amount of baking soda applied with a soft toothbrush or nailbrush – spend about three minutes brushing each nail and wash off. Many transparent nail hardeners can double up as clear varnish. And do use a base coat before applying colour and a top coat if you've got the time, the nail colour will last much longer and be resistant to chipping.

Our nails should be healthy because of how we've improved our diet. The nail itself should be smooth and shiny and pink, almost translucent.

> Whilst we're looking at feet, let's look at your shoes. Your feet will be going through their own metamorphosis.

## Not-to-be-forgotten feet

When we're heavy, our feet struggle to cope with the change in their centre of gravity. They splay and broaden, and ligaments and tendons become strained – not to mention metatarsals.

sometime soon

Basic foot-care is vital for us to feel good — and it requires a little bit more effort than just washing regularly and cutting your toenails. Skin-softening and rough skin removal products, a brisk session with a pumice stone and moisturiser, and a bit of cuticle attention can work wonders — and the results are often instantly visible too.

Whilst we're looking at feet, let's look at your shoes. Your feet will be going through their own metamorphosis, the same as everywhere else on you. They may begin to look a little slimmer and shoes seem less pinched. If you've not been able to wear strappy styles because the straps haven't been long enough to fit your foot's broadness, then a whole new experience awaits! And when you're ready for a heel, give it a try. A heel gives you height, slims the leg and gives you a definite sway to the hips.

If you've always been a 'flattie' then, yes, you've always been comfortable, but often thin-soled flats are not as supportive as shoes with a small heel. It's going to take time to get used to a heel, and those calf muscles will complain, but if there was ever a time to start making those style changes, then it's now. However old the frock, it can be updated with an amazing pair of shoes. Practise indoors before you launch yourself outside; give yourself a chance to learn to walk with confidence, then off you go.

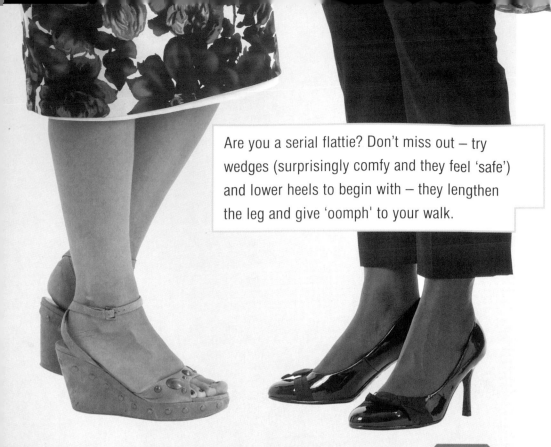

Are you a serial flattie? Don't miss out — try wedges (surprisingly comfy and they feel 'safe') and lower heels to begin with — they lengthen the leg and give 'oomph' to your walk.

When you are exercising, it's vital to have your foot and ankle supported properly with correctly fitting sports shoes. Start with some cross-trainers, that is, trainers that suit a variety of purposes over a mixture of terrains. You should have a thumb's width of room at the end of your longest toe, because your feet may swell by half a size during strenuous use. The shoe should hold your foot securely around the arch and instep, and at the heel with little or no slipping. Wear specialist sports socks which are thicker and will minimise slippage and rubbing, and take out the standard issue insole and buy a replacement insole straight away - it will be thicker and more durable.

sometime soon

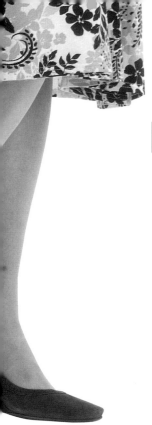

## More massage

Are you hooked on massage by now? It can become something of an addiction!

Try this technique yourself at home to benefit your legs and feet – especially if your day is mostly sedentary. Sit on the bed and use your thumbs to apply light pressure in a circulatory motion under the arches of your feet. (Hope you're not ticklish!) Continue up to the ankle bones and up the backs of the calves. Move on to the knees. Use your thumbs on the front, then on the sensitive backs of the knees, curl your fingers up into a fist shape and knead gently on up the inside of your thigh. Knead and pinch gently the tops of the thighs to stimulate the area and get things working.

A daily pressure-point facial massage using cleanser, moisturiser or a facial oil will help reduce puffiness; it will also promote circulation and, if done last thing at night, will give a nice healthy glow by the next morning. It's a simple technique, easily learned, and involves pressing a line of imaginary dots a centimetre apart. Work from the centre of your forehead near the hairline outwards; the centre of your eyebrows and outwards; from either side of your nose, over the cheekbones and outwards; from the corners of the mouth up to the cheekbones; from the sides of the nose down to the chin, and a gentle pinch along the jawline using both thumbs and forefingers from the chin to just under the ears. Gently drum the skin with all fingers to finish.

## Slimming make-up tips

Our faces are worth spending time on, whether we like our looks or not. However pleased we are with our changing bodies, we often forget that what most people notice is our faces; they'll visually take in our whole head and neckline at one fell swoop before unconsciously letting their eyes drift to our bodies. And perhaps there are bits of our bodies we'd still rather people didn't look at? How can we keep people looking where we want them to look? By presenting the best possible 'face' you can.

Did you take advantage of a department-store make-up makeover, as suggested in the previous section to kickstart your style makeover? If so, you'll have seen that make-up doesn't have to be slapped on to be noticeable; there are many subtle products that give a very natural effect, but present a more finished, more polished and groomed look to match your new, more polished and groomed wardrobe. Minimal effort and coverage requires a light face base (always with an SPF factor). After you've cleansed and moisturised in the morning, apply a matt base with a little loose powder to set it. This is the speediest and most foolproof method to give the skin an even tone and disguise any redness. Decide on either lips or eyes as the main focus – both is a look for evening only. If the emphasis is on the lips then play down the eyes. Use a soft shadow pencil, complementary to your eye colour, along the base of the upper lashes and smudge it with your little finger. Then follow with a brush of

sometime soon

# However pleased we are with our changing bodies, we often forget that what most people notice is our faces.

mascara. A little make-up for the eyebrows will also help frame the eyes and make the whole face come more alive. Pencil or powder colours can be used to define the shape and fill in any gaps. Don't over do it and certainly do not try to alter your natural shape brow with excessive use of product, as it will almost certainly look false.

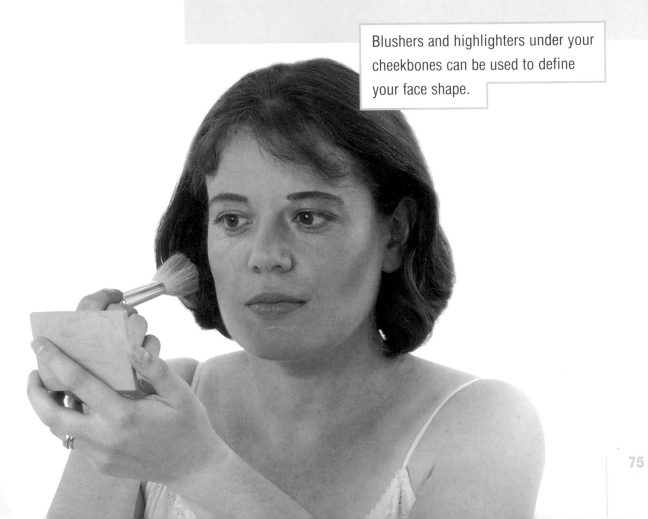

Blushers and highlighters under your cheekbones can be used to define your face shape.

To complement our new, slimmer bodies, there are a couple of make-up tips which slim the face. Try using blusher and bronzer colours on the inner brow, under the cheekbone and at the jawline. Imagine you're sketching a monkeynut-shape inside a circle – you're creating shadows to elongate the face. To slim the nose, a light brush of colour down each side, topped with an illuminating product on the tip, well blended in, will have a slimming effect. Illuminating products will have a similar effect applied on the chin, on the throat and  – if wearing a V-neck – down to the bosom. It's to create a central 'light' that hopefully by now is almost mesmerising!

> One of the most blissful and defining moments at this stage of weight loss is when we find we have a drawer full of baggy knickers!

## Firmer new foundations

If you can notice your clothing becoming baggier, then you'll surely notice the same with underwear. Bras aren't digging in and, rather than being on the last possible notch, you can move one or two notches up and perk yourself up in an instant by tightening the shoulder straps. But there's a dangerous precipice you can fall into here – what's baggy today might be detrimental to your bosom tomorrow. Suddenly having space within the individual cups isn't doing your breasts any good; chances are they're not as well supported as they once were and could be straining muscle and delicate tissue. You thought the danger time for stretch marks was when

sometime soon

you were putting on weight; in fact, the same applies when losing weight. Your bosom needs supporting all along the way!

Now's the time to get measured for new lingerie. Ideally, a bra wardrobe should include a white, a black, a nude, a pretty and a sports style. Use a store's bra-fitting service, as outlined in the first section of this book, and be measured for all styles while you can. There's no obligation to buy everything you try on.

However tempting novelty bras are — dressy styles as opposed to working styles — remember that this is another one of those transitory items which may not fit in a few months' time. This is to improve what you have right now, to get you to the next stage; don't blow your budget, but do go for universal-use, plainer-quality styles rather than frippery. And, of course, bras stretch and lose a certain amount of elasticity through wear and washing, so buy the bra that fits you best on the loosest hook; as it stretches, you'll be able to make it tighter and thus ensure a perfect fit as time passes.

## It's not all pants

One of the most blissful and defining moments at this stage of weight-loss is when we find we have a drawer full of baggy knickers! When they get too baggy, ditch them without a second glance. But we're still in full-pant land, perhaps verging on briefs, shorts and French knickers. Have patience, things are getting more exciting every day, but we're not quite ready for thongs, low-rise styles or strings — yet!

Fashions come and go in all garment departments - even knickers. Whilst the invention of the thong made all big pants seem old-fashioned, we're finally turning our backs on these skimpy styles. A thong avoids a visible panty line, but it's often uncomfortable, rather brash, and can even become a health hazard as it may encourage yeast infections. Big, Bridget Jones-style pants are now swiftly increasing in popularity once more. When it comes to lingerie, it seems that comfort rules all.

Control pants are fully recommended for this 'in-between' stage if the sizing is available — and please don't be despondent if you're not quite there yet; it's something to look forward to. Control pants have become universally known as 'magic' garments. They rely on seamless fabric technology, resemble fine cycling shorts, and hold in and smooth out lumps and bumps, if you're beginning to feel that a bit of waist or hips could be revealed. Some styles can even, with padding, create 'lift and shape' — but maybe that's something for the future!

Control underwear can smooth out lumps and bumps.

# sometime soon

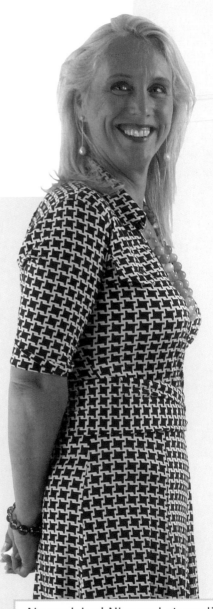

Sales of control underwear are on the increase! Waist-shaping corsets, bum hold-ups, hold-you-in tights and miracle swimsuits are all recent additions to our wardrobes. It's decades since we, as a nation, wore roll-ons or panty-girdles, but modern equivalents are gaining huge popularity. They're ideal for that special outfit we still find a bit of a squeeze.

## Accessories add oomph

If you had an uninteresting dark corner in your house, you'd add a pretty light and a bunch of flowers to breathe life into it, yes? Similarly, your greatly pared-down wardrobe, with its newly altered, second-time-around garments could probably do with a bit of a boost. Even if they're not all grey, verging on black, tones, chances are you could do with a bit of colour and texture to lift the overall effect. However dated or dull a wardrobe, it can be brought bang up to date by investing in a whole variety of accessories.

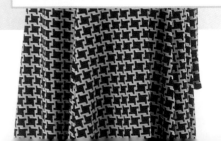
Abracadabra! Nice and streamlined!

Every season there's a new 'now' colour or 'now' fabric. Scour the latest fashion pages for advance notice of what's arriving in the stores. Accessory departments and specialist accessory stores are thriving today because, as a nation, we're rather obsessed by shoes, handbags, scarves and jewellery.

## Scarves and brooches

If you normally go for tonal colours, try a clashing colour – or vice versa. A long, chunky necklace on top will add interest to your face, neck and décolleté. Remember to focus in on this area to divert attention from the still-to-be-worked-on zones! Feature brooches and fabric corsages add interest to a lapel on a plain jacket, especially if toning with a scarf or at the neckline to draw attention to the cleavage.

## Necklaces, bracelets and rings

It doesn't matter if jewellery is 'real' or fake, it adds a finishing touch to most outfits. There are some rules. Don't wear different styles of jewellery all at the same time. The 'mix' will be misleading and messy if there isn't an overriding theme. A chunky necklace requires a chunky bracelet and ring; fine chains perhaps require a feature stone or crystal to add interest. Gold and silver doesn't always mix unless it's wildly mixed, perhaps with copper too; but bling can often be blinging awful! Think of jewellery as wearable art, which is

Don't create a messy mix of styles; it looks 'thrown together'!

What to wear when you are losing weight
sometime soon

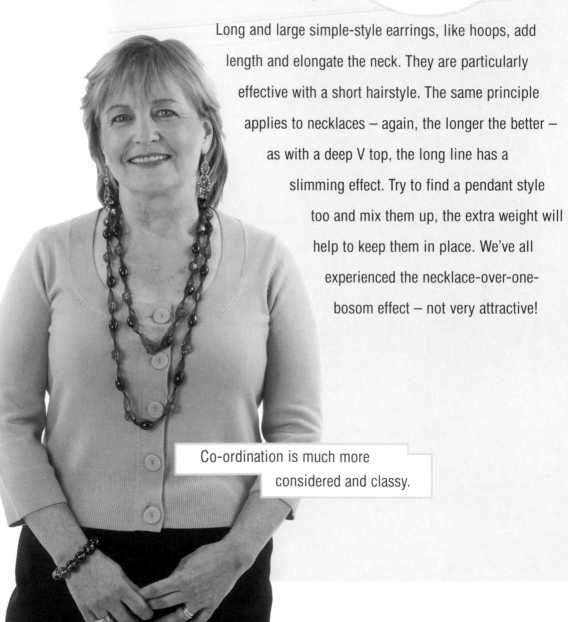

accentuating a colour you're already wearing on a top, or on your eyes or even in your hair. Imagine the warmth of amber next to chestnut hair; a strong fashion colour against a dark top for drama; a selection of crystals to accentuate a delicate sheer lip gloss.

Long and large simple-style earrings, like hoops, add length and elongate the neck. They are particularly effective with a short hairstyle. The same principle applies to necklaces – again, the longer the better – as with a deep V top, the long line has a slimming effect. Try to find a pendant style too and mix them up, the extra weight will help to keep them in place. We've all experienced the necklace-over-one-bosom effect – not very attractive!

Co-ordination is much more considered and classy.

Bracelets and bangles add colour and texture and look terrific piled high whilst wearing a three-quarter sleeve top. All eyes will be diverted on to the bangles, away from 'difficult' upper arms! Same goes for rings. Wear chunky styles, in twos and threes to add character and help with proportion – but watch that they don't look tight and squeezed.

# Keep up the great work

- ✓ Keep on weighing . . .

- ✓ Keep on measuring . . .

- ✓ Keep on noticing new trends and applying them in sensible stages . . .

This is a transitory period and perhaps the most exciting!

sometime soon

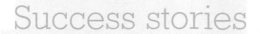

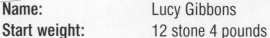

| | |
|---|---|
| **Name:** | Lucy Gibbons |
| **Start weight:** | 12 stone 4 pounds |
| **Weight now:** | 9 stone 2 pounds |
| **Clothes size before:** | 16 |
| **Clothes size now:** | 10 to 12 |
| **Meeting:** | Sedgley, West Midlands |

I started worrying about my weight probably in my teens, when I was bigger than most of my friends. I've always loved food and was brought up to finish everything on my plate. As I grew older I tried several diets, but I found them confusing to follow and difficult to stick to, so I always quickly lost motivation.

At university in Birmingham, I fell for a handsome gymnastics instructor, Lee. Contented and happy, in a loving, secure relationship, the pounds crept on. It was when I looked at photos of myself on our summer holiday together in 2002 that I decided I really had to do something about my weight. I went along to a local Weight Watchers meeting with Lee's mum and was horrified to find that I had reached 12 stone 4 pounds!

I followed the *POINTS* programme and was delighted that I managed to get down to 10 stone 7 pounds. I gradually stopped attending the meetings during my last year at university. But when I began work as a primary school teacher, I was careful to keep on track. I kept my eye on the Weight Watchers programme and bought a Weight Watchers cookbook to use at home.

Then, totally out of the blue, Lee went down on one knee during a thunderstorm and proposed. It was very dramatic, and of course, I said yes! I became determined to get down to my goal weight in time for my wedding, and I went with my friend Laura to her Weight Watchers meeting in Sedgley. This time I tried the NoCount food plan, and with the help of my wonderfully supportive leader, Anne, I dropped those final few pounds. Now I've just had the final fitting for my wedding dress – I am so proud of the results of all my hard work. If I can do it, anyone can.

# Success stories

**Name:** Claire Brennan
**Start weight:** 15 stone 8 pounds
**Weight now:** 12 stone 4 pounds
**Clothes size before:** 22
**Clothes size now:** 16 to 18
**Meeting:** Holborn, Central London

When I looked at photos of myself on an evening with friends in November 2000, I couldn't believe how big I was. I'd been kidding myself that I carried my weight well and didn't look that bad. I was ashamed of what my friends must think of me – and no wonder I was single!

The next week, I joined Weight Watchers. I loved the idea of being able to eat what you want so long as it's within your daily allowance. By New Year's Eve I'd lost a stone and felt fantastic. With my new-found confidence, I went out feeling great. I had a fantastic time, and met a gorgeous man – Charlie.

Over the next 18 months, I got down to 11 stone 6 pounds. It was amazing to be able to go into a high-street shop and buy something other than shoes and jewellery. However, getting engaged and moving in with Charlie meant that I began to indulge in lots of meals out and takeaways in. I kept going to Weight Watchers meetings, but the weight crept back on until, a year after our wedding, I tipped the 13 stone mark once more. I didn't feel attractive or sexy – which isn't great as a newly-wed! I forced myself to take a good look at what I was really eating, and I also joined the gym and made myself go three times a week. I began helping my Weight Watchers leader at meetings, which motivated me to stay focussed, as an inspiration to others.

So now I am lighter and feeling great again. I went shopping recently for my summer wardrobe and it was just wonderful to be able to buy colourful, womanly, non-tentlike clothes. I feel fitter, more attractive and far more confident than I ever have. Weight Watchers has really changed my life.

**Claire's style tip:** If a top is too short and your tummy is poking out then try layering with a longer vest top underneath.

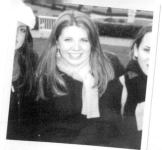

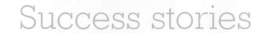

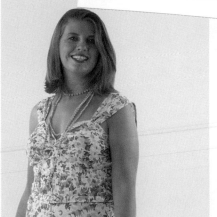

| | |
|---|---|
| **Name:** | Amanda Shipp |
| **Start weight:** | 14 stone 7 pounds |
| **Weight now:** | 12 stone 12 pounds |
| **Weight lost:** | 1 stone 9 pounds |
| **Clothes size before:** | 16 to 18 |
| **Clothes size now:** | 14 to 16 |
| **Meeting:** | London, SW12 |

I had never been one hundred percent happy with my size, but always made up excuses not to do anything about it. However, in November 2003, I met a long-lost friend who had always been a similar size and shape to me. She had lost lots of weight and looked fantastic! She explained that she had joined Weight Watchers and told me how easy it was to follow the *POINTS* system. So I decided – no more excuses! It was time to focus on losing weight properly.

I joined Weight Watchers, and the first weigh-in shock gave me all the motivation I needed. As the pounds came off, I realised how limited I had previously been for clothes. I began to express myself by trying a variety of new styles and colours, enjoying the freedom of choosing from a wider range of shops. After I lost my first stone, I also started to run. Previously, I considered myself 'just not made for running', but I started slowly (just 10 minutes at a time), built up gradually, and recently ran a half-marathon, have joined a ladies' football team, and am contemplating the London Marathon next year!

I know that I need the support from Weight Watchers meetings and weekly weigh-ins, together with my structured fitness goals, to keep me on track with my *POINTS* allowance and with my exercising. Being open about Weight Watchers has also helped – instead of urging me to have another glass of wine or a pudding, people praise me when I hold back. I feel fitter and have more energy than ever before – best of all, it's now my turn to be complimented when I run into people I haven't seen for a few years . . .

**Amanda's style tip:** I find that a pair of heels work wonders on any outfit and always makes you feel slimmer.

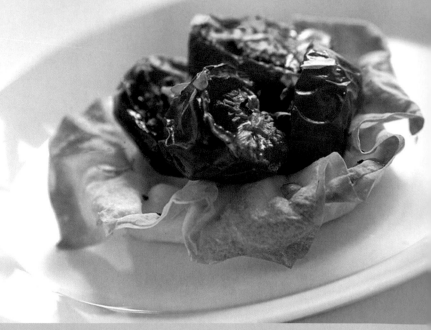

# Recipes for success

**More quick and tasty recipes to keep you on track.**

## Oven-roasted tomato tartlets

1 kg (2 lb 4 oz) plum tomatoes
1 teaspoon salt
8 sheets of filo pastry
2 tablespoons olive oil
2 tablespoons fresh basil leaves, torn (optional)
freshly ground black pepper

makes **8**   **1** POINTS VALUE   Per serving   **120** cals   **V**

- Preparation time 15 minutes.
- Cooking time 1$\frac{1}{2}$ hours.
- Freezing recommended for the roasted tomatoes only.
- 10 **POINTS** values per recipe

Slow roasting tomatoes brings out their wonderful rich flavour.

1   Preheat the oven to Gas Mark 2/150°C/300°F.

2   Slice the tomatoes in half horizontally and arrange cut-side up on a cooling rack. Lift the cooling rack over a baking sheet and then sprinkle the salt over the tomatoes.

3   Roast the tomatoes in the oven for 1 hour, until they are beginning to dry out a little.

4   After the tomatoes have cooked, increase the oven temperature to Gas Mark 5/190°C/ 375°F. Cut each sheet of filo pastry in half, brush with olive oil and sandwich two halves together. Press into 8 individual tartlet tins scrunching up the edges with your fingers so the pastry fits into the tins. Brush the insides of the tartlet cases with any remaining olive oil and place a crumpled piece of foil into each one. Bake for 15 minutes, until the pastry is crisp and golden.

5   Carefully remove the pastry cases from the tins and fill with the roasted tomato halves.

6   Scatter each tartlet with a little torn basil, if using, and a generous grinding of black pepper.

**Cook's note:** It's better to tear fresh basil rather than chop it, since this prevents it from bruising.

# Cod fillets pizza-style

4 x 100 g (3¹/2 oz) cod fillets

225 g (8 oz) canned chopped tomatoes

2 tablespoons tomato purée

50 g (1³/4 oz) pitted black olives, halved

2 tablespoons fresh basil, torn

25 g (1 oz) freshly grated parmesan

salt and freshly ground black pepper

serves 4

**2** POINTS VALUE

Per serving **120** cals

- Preparation time 10 minutes.
- Cooking time 25 minutes.
- Freezing recommended.
- 8 *POINTS* values per recipe

Serve with freshly cooked vegetables or a side salad.

1   Rinse the cod steaks and pat dry with absorbent kitchen paper. Line a roasting tin with non-stick baking parchment and lift the fish steaks into the tin. Preheat the oven to Gas Mark 5/190°C/375°F.

2   Mix together the chopped tomatoes, tomato purée, olives, basil and seasoning and spread equal amounts over each cod steak. Sprinkle the parmesan over the top and bake for 20 to 25 minutes, until the fish is cooked through and the cheese has melted.

**Cook's note:** A crushed garlic clove can be added to the tomatoes if liked.

# Cock-a-leekie soup

1 medium chicken leg quarter, skinned

1 chicken stock cube

50 g (1³/4 oz) pearl barley

1 bay leaf

2 onions, sliced

2 leeks, sliced

1 carrot, chopped

2 tablespoons chopped fresh parsley

salt and freshly ground black pepper

serves 4

**1½** POINTS VALUE

Per serving **155** cals

- Preparation time 10 minutes.
- Cooking time 1 hour.
- Freezing recommended.
- 6¹/2 *POINTS* values per recipe

Simmering a chicken quarter with the vegetables gives this soup a great flavour. It's inexpensive and very nourishing too.

1   Put the chicken portion into a large saucepan and add 1.2 litres (2 pints) of cold water and the stock cube. Add the pearl barley and bay leaf, and bring up to the boil. Reduce the heat and simmer gently, partially covered, for 30 minutes.

2   Add the onions, leeks and carrot to the saucepan and continue to cook for about 20 minutes until the vegetables are tender and the pearl barley is cooked.

3   Lift the chicken portion from the saucepan, cool slightly, then remove all the meat from the bones. Chop the meat and return to the saucepan with the parsley.

4   Remove the bay leaf, reheat the soup and season to taste. Ladle into warmed bowls.

## Open-topped bacon and tomato toastie

1 medium slice of wholemeal bread

1 teaspoon low-fat spread

1 rasher lean back bacon

1 small tomato, thinly sliced

2 to 3 red onion rings

1 low-fat cheese slice

salt and freshly ground black pepper

serves 1 · 4 POINTS VALUE · 255 cals

- Preparation and cooking time 20 minutes.
- Freezing not recommended.
- A speedy lunchtime snack, guaranteed to fill you up.
- 4 **POINTS** values per recipe

1 Lightly toast the bread on both sides and spread with low fat spread.

2 Grill the bacon slice until just crispy and lift onto the toast. Arrange the tomato slices over the bacon with the onion rings. Top with the cheese slice and season.

## Vegetable noodles with ginger and soy

250 g (9 oz) medium egg noodles

1 tablespoon sunflower oil

2.5 cm (1 inch) root ginger, grated

1 garlic clove, crushed

175 g (6 oz) carrots, cut into thin sticks

2 celery stalks, trimmed and sliced

150 g (5½ oz) mushrooms, sliced

175 g (6 oz) courgettes, trimmed and cut into sticks

100 g (3½ oz) mange-tout peas, trimmed

100 g (3½ oz) baby corn, trimmed and halved

6 spring onions, trimmed and sliced

3 tablespoons soy sauce

1 tablespoon medium sherry

  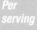  

serves 4 · 3½ POINTS VALUE · Per serving 340 cals · V

- Preparation and cooking time 25 minutes.
- Freezing recommended.
- 15 **POINTS** values per recipe

1 Place the noodles in a bowl and pour boiling water over. Leave to stand for 10 minutes.

2 Heat the oil in a large pan or wok and stir-fry the ginger, garlic, carrots, celery, mushrooms, courgettes, mange-tout peas and corn for 5 minutes.

3 Drain the noodles and toss into the vegetables with the spring onions, soy sauce and sherry. Cook for a further 2 to 3 minutes.

**Cook's note:** When you buy a piece of root ginger, keep what you don't use in the freezer so you can just grate a little as and when you need it.

# Mustard mash

1 kg (2 lb 4 oz) potatoes
150 ml (5 fl oz) skimmed milk
50 g (1 3/4 oz) hot English mustard
salt and freshly ground black pepper

serves 4
3 POINTS VALUE
Per serving
225 cals
V

- Preparation time 15 minutes.
- Cooking time 30–45 minutes
- Freezing not recommended.
- 11 1/2 **POINTS** values per recipe

Simple mashed potato is one of the best comfort foods.

1   Put the potatoes into a large pan of boiling salted water and boil for at least 30 minutes until tender when you insert the point of a knife into the largest one.

2   Drain and, holding each hot potato in a tea towel, peel them using the back of a knife. Return to the pan and mash them with a hand masher. Do not be tempted to use a food processor as you will end up with a sticky mess!

3   Add the milk, mustard and seasoning. Stir together then serve.

# Apple and cinnamon French toast

1 cooking apple
2 eggs
300 ml (1/2 pint) skimmed milk
1 tablespoon caster sugar
1/2 teaspoon ground cinnamon
4 thick slices of two-day-old white or wholemeal bread
low-fat cooking spray
1 teaspoon demerara sugar

serves 4
3 POINTS VALUE
Per serving
200 cals
V

- Preparation time 20 minutes.
- Cooking time 15 minutes.
- Freezing not recommended.
- 12 1/2 **POINTS** values per recipe

Serve with a spoonful of creme fraîche if you wish, but don't forget to add the extra **POINTS** values.

1   Peel the cooking apple and core. Dice finely and place in a pan with 1 tablespoon of water. Cover and cook gently until pulpy. Allow to cool.

2   Place the eggs, milk, sugar, cinnamon and cooked apple in a food processor and blend until smooth. Transfer to a shallow dish.

3   Cut each piece of bread in half and dip in the apple and egg mixture, leaving it to soak in for 2 to 3 minutes per side.

4   Spray a non-stick frying-pan with low-fat cooking spray and heat. Cook the French toast slices for 2 to 3 minutes per side until golden. Serve 2 pieces per person, sprinkled with a little demerara sugar.

e the future

the future th

Part 3

These are the final stages in the life and the usefulness of the treasured weight-loss and measurement chart next to the wardrobe! It may be a little dog-eared now, but you're now pretty much near your goal. It's a magnificent result and one that deserves a pat on the back. To have relieved your body of those unwanted pounds is a wonderful thing; but now we have to recognise that we might gain some weight back if we don't continue with the positive lifestyle changes we have made. Attending meetings regularly, and if necessary creating another chart where our target remains level, may help to stay on track.

We've all been on different journeys and have had different goals; we may now be a size 14 where we once were a 20, we may now be a 20 where we once were a 32, we may now be a 16 instead of a 24. It could be a much 'smaller' result like a 12 instead of a 16, but it's still a new shape. We may sometimes feel like a stranger (a gorgeous one!) that greets us in the mirror each morning. At almost goal weight, it's vital to take your measurements once more and revisit those clothes-sizing charts. You may well want to try on styles you've not tried before, and knowledge is power!

We may sometimes feel like a stranger (a gorgeous one!)

# What's your style?

For however long it's taken to reach almost goal weight, you've been promising to give your wardrobe a complete re-hash, re-invention and revitalisation. Now, finally, you have a new, leaner, fitter body to celebrate – and the fashion world is your oyster.

It's quite probable that you are now saying 'I have nothing to wear' and it's true. But where do you go from here with your wardrobe? However long your journey has taken, along the way you've been noticing fashion more and how it evolves and changes. What was 'in' might now be 'out'; or even be back 'in' again. Fashion is notoriously fickle.

Ask yourself some questions:

✓ **Do you like and suit what's currently in vogue?** Or are you struggling to find something that is really you?

✓ **Have you got a strong sense of identity?** Does your character shine through and is it enhanced by your choice of clothing?

✓ **Do you tend to buy classic styles in timeless fabrics?** Or are you more interested in following the trends every season? Are you happy to buy fast-fashion, wear it, and quickly ditch it?

✓ **Are you stuck in a style era?** From the 80s – big shoulder pads and big hair? From the 90s – mad for labels? Or more recent Boho?

✓ **Do you dress to suit your age?** Your way of life?

There are no right or wrong answers. One word is important here: improvement. The long and often laborious journey that we've undertaken has been one of improvement, of our health and our well-being. There's been a physical change and we're making the very best of ourselves. We look better now than we've ever done and to take it one step further, through clothing, we're going to enhance our image even further.

## Perfect proportions

You may want to want to choose clothes to show off all your new 'best bits' at once, but this may not work from a fashion point of view. An outfit needs just one focal point, not several. For instance, a long backless dress requires the focus to fall on the beautiful line of the spine; to see knees at the same time will spoil the sophistication of the overall look. Add emphasis to the bit you want others to notice, but let the rest of the outfit work as a blank canvas to highlight it.

Even though we now know our size blindfolded, remember that the design of each garment we are contemplating buying dictates its size. It may say size 16, 14 or 12, but if it's a fitted design then it is a shaped garment and may not be flattering. A semi-fitted garment follows the figure shape but hints at it rather than hugs it. A traditional fit, which usually doesn't warrant a special mention, is usually more straight-sided. A loose fit is self-explanatory: this will be a drop-shoulder design with a hip measurement to mirror the top, or it will be a slightly-flared design which fits at the shoulder but flows over the hip. Some garments carry warnings if shrinkage is going to be noticeable; take it as a tip to buy a larger size.

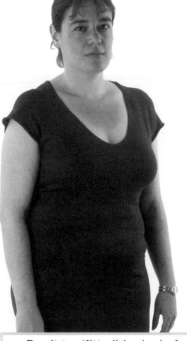

Don't try 'fitted' looks before you're ready for them.

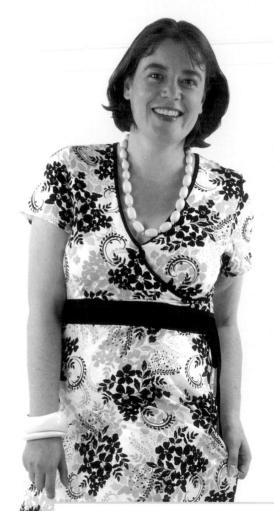

Choose styles that 'fit' in areas you're OK about and 'skim' those you're not.

At the end of your journey, have you uncovered a pear-shape? Accentuate your gorgeous waist with fitted jackets, tops and dresses. If you have achieved a perfect bottom, too, then celebrate with a pencil skirt – if not, an A-line or full skirt will further emphasise the definition of your waist. If you still prefer to hide a little, try shirt-dresses and tunics – unbuttoned, with a close-fitting T-shirt underneath to show your flatter tum.

## Amber for 'proceed with caution'

Now we can expose our flesh. Don't be shocked – we're not going to strip off with gay abandon. We're going to experiment thoughtfully and carefully. Here are the styles to be wary of:

- ✓ **Strappy tops** – they really only look very good on firmly toned arms: it's a fact.

- ✓ **Midriff styles** – unless you've developed a washboard stomach, or are very young, leave well alone.

- ✓ **Short shorts** – by all means wear on the beach, and in town experiment with city-shorts styles which are longer and more tailored than holiday shorts.

When it comes to fabrics, remember that some can actually make you look heavier and add bulk. For instance, tweed adds bulk – and also, in larger sizes, can look rather frumpy however trendy the style. Velvet relies on the light for its sumptuous effect, but over some of our still-present lumps and bumps the fabric will just emphasise exactly what we're trying to hide! And affordable leather, unless on small sizes, can look like a cheap sofa. Yes, that does sound harsh, but it's the truth.

Beware of fabrics that give the illusion of bulk.

Wear potentially tricky fabrics in the correct proportions and it's a completely different effect.

## Green for 'GO, GO, GO!'

Now we're almost at goal weight, these are styles to try which you may not have thought about before:

✓ **Clingier styles in clingier fabrics** – fluid jersey emphasises not just your figure but also your body movement.

✓ **See-through fabrics in demure styles** – try layering transparent and gauzy and lace fabrics, or wear transparent over fabulous underwear that's designed to be seen (such as a vintage camisole or a corset-style bodice). With their glimpse and hint of flesh, these are so much sexier than overt exposure.

✓ **Colour, prints, texture and embroidery** – what may have seemed over-fussy, loud and enlarging before can now be worn to its best advantage, looking feminine and fun.

✓ **Louder and more interesting tights and stockings** – our legs can be more of a focal point than ever before. If your legs are less than perfect in texture or appearance rather than shape just make your choice from 60-denier styles. You've been hiding those pins for far too long.

✓ **All those bras which were only available in smaller sizes** – to show off our newly emerged collarbones and what seems like a longer neck. The décolleté and shoulder area can become a new major focal point. Where before, straps used to strain (we've all suffered the ugly

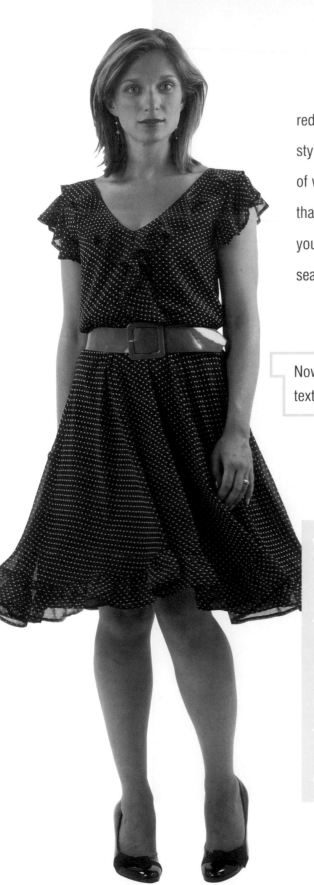

red strap-mark syndrome), we can start to look at styles with 'feature' straps in delicate lace, many of which are designed to be seen. (Don't forget that white undies show through white clothes. If you want 'invisible', nude shades in smooth seam-free styles are the best.)

Now you can experiment with prints and textures — they can look feminine and fun.

What may have seemed over-fussy, loud and enlarging before can now be worn to its best advantage.

Don't be fooled into thinking that a tan has a slimming effect - it makes no difference. However, if you have very pale skin, a tan may make you feel more attractive. The only really safe way to get a tan is out of a bottle - but don't overdo it. And don't think you can get away with just applying it to the face and neck, or you will leave tell-tale signs such as the hands and ankles not matching, and a bizarre tidemark if your neckline slips! For a special occasion, why not invest in having fake tan applied by a professional at a beauty salon?

## The ultimate shopping experience

It's the stuff of dreams isn't it? Everything we couldn't have before is now so very available, and if we've been saving for this special day, we can buy what we want! But beware — we must learn to cope with this new-found shopping freedom. We used to buy clothes just because they fitted, rather than because they suited us or because they were what we needed. Now we must get out of this habit, or we'll overspend on the entirely inappropriate. We can be picky, and have the choice to buy or not to buy. This new, fun feeling will make your heart sing!

Now our choice of store is much wider than before. We can go where we like, according to our budget. A sensible option is to buy an item or two

We used to
buy clothes just
because they
fitted, rather
than because
they suited us.

every week. Learn to live with the items and mix them with other things in your wardrobe before buying the next piece. We often think of fashion as fast because the majority of us rush around the shops at the weekend, when everyone else does. But who says that fashion-buying has to be fast and frenetic? Try visiting the high street on a Monday morning (take a day off – you deserve it, you've got something to celebrate!) and it's a totally different world – the rails are tidy, stocked to the brim with the morning's deliveries, and there's often not a soul in sight . . . bliss! Popular items will, of course, disappear very quickly indeed. But go at your own pace and reflect peacefully on the fact that you don't want to wear what everyone else is wearing anyway!

## Create your own clothing concept

We've arrived at this day because of all our fantastic efforts. And we have a slimmed-down wardrobe, as well as a slimmed-down bod, because we've learned to throw things away rather than hoard. Now we've come this far, it would be a shame not to plan to get the perfect end result for our new image. What we should aim for in the ideal stylish new wardrobe is a mix of the core classic basics together with some highly individual pieces and a few fashion pieces to acknowledge the trends of the season, all put together to create our individual personal look.

Remember the personal shopper? If you didn't try this service before, now is the time. And even if you did, it's a great time to revisit your personal shopper. He or she may remember you – part of this highly individual service requires the meticulous logging of personal details such as your likes and dislikes, your measurements and colouring. But this time around, your measurements and body shape will have changed. Your hair colour may even have changed. And thus begins a whole new round of tips and trying-on. Let's face it, there'll be even more fun to be had now with trying on completely unfamiliar styles, patterns and colourways. Your choice is so much wider.

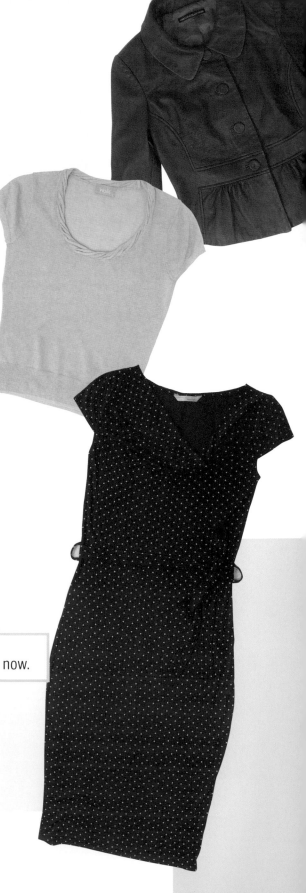

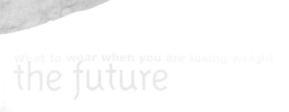

Dresses and 'softs' are going to be part of our wardrobes now.

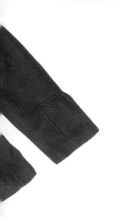

So what are we aiming for? However much fashion seasons and trends change, some core items are always necessary:

- ✓ outerwear – coats, macs and jackets
- ✓ smart tailoring, or smart separates to resemble suiting for work or more formal occasions
- ✓ good basics like white t-shirts and shirts, perfect-fitting jeans
- ✓ casual and comfortable pieces for lounging and adventuring
- ✓ dresses and 'softs' – for days when you want to dress up
- ✓ party pieces to add oomph.

Let's face it, there'll be even more fun to be had now with trying on completely unfamiliar styles, patterns and colourways. Your choice is so much wider.

Are you on the tall side, newly slim, now with a lean body shape? Ironically, you may need to emphasise a bit of the shape you've tried so hard to lose! Bias-cut dresses help to give the illusion of curves - you're the only figure-shape that can successfully get away with them. You'll suit low-rise trousers and jeans to accentuate your hips. You can show off your shapely arms and legs in sleeveless and short styles. And don't forget dramatic styles such as backless dresses.

## Finding the perfect pair of jeans

Jeans are a basic and a classic. They go with everything and can be dressed up or down to suit almost every occasion. Jeans are very much a style statement and, now that we've 'arrived', we simply have to have some!

There are more denim brands than you can shake a stick at and jeans are a part of any mainstream retailer's own collection too. Like any staple fashion item, jeans have become the subject of whim and change with the trend of the season. Jeans aficionados are concerned with features such as original copper rivets, and left-weave and rare Japanese denim fabric. But what we should concentrate on is simply the fit. This may mean trying on every pair you can find and not bothering about the label; it also depends on your budget!

 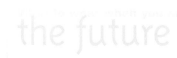

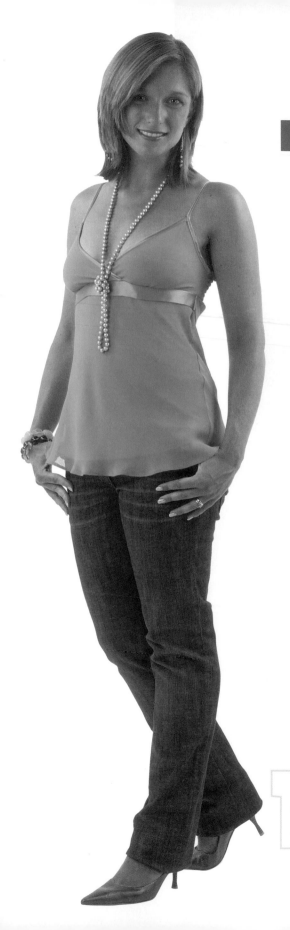

## Colour and cut

If you've been out of the jeans market for a while, jeans terminology will be unfamiliar:

✓ The darker the denim, the more slimming the effect. The whiter the fade on the jeans, the wider the look. If you must have fade, go for a subtle 'handwash' effect down the centre of the leg.

✓ High-waisted styles act as a corset and are a godsend if your tummy hasn't yet lost its roundness or sag.

✓ Stretch jeans are a modern miracle – but too tight and they'll cling to less-than-perfect places. Try to go for a skimming effect rather than a cling, it's far more flattering.

✓ Straight-leg, sometimes called cigarette, are often the most flattering cut. They help elongate the leg. The smartest-looking jean, they can be teamed successfully with smarter tailoring or a crisp white shirt.

Darker non-decorative jeans are the most versatile dressed 'up' or 'down' and therefore the best investment.

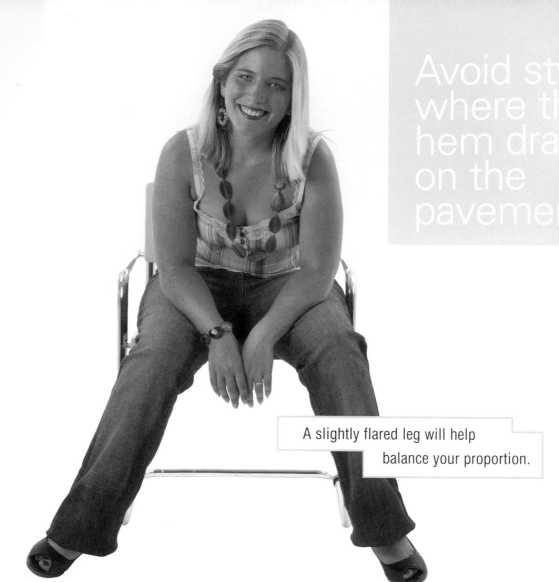

Avoid styles where the hem drags on the pavement!

A slightly flared leg will help balance your proportion.

Alternatively, because they are so plain, they can be teamed with a more dramatic-shaped top like a trapeze-style or a kimono-sleeve, and certainly more flamboyant boots, shoes or sandals.

✓ Bootcut are snug around the thigh but flare out slightly from the knee downwards. If your bottom is still a little over-heavy, the slightly flared leg will help balance your proportion – but avoid styles where the hem drags on the pavement!

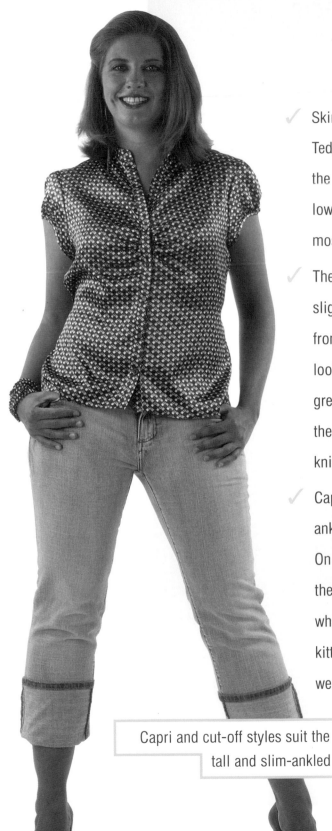

✓ Skinny are, well, skinny – a modern version of Teddyboy drainpipes – and are very firmly for the matchstick kind of leg. They're usually very low waisted – and not the most flattering for most of us.

✓ The boy-fit is snug on the hips, but with a slightly baggy thigh, one grade of bagginess up from 'skimming'. It's a casual weekend style that looks like they're borrowed from a boyfriend – great with sneakers and a vest top to counteract the boyishness, but equally good with luxurious knits or fitted tops and a girly heel.

✓ Capri or cut-off styles only work with slim ankles and on those tall enough to carry it off. On others, the cut-off proportion foreshortens the body. They are perfect for the gamine girl when worn with delicate flat pumps – or try a kitten-heel sandal, or a straw or rope holiday wedge-style shoe.

Capri and cut-off styles suit the tall and slim-ankled amongst us!

Because jeans are such a design classic it's perhaps wise to own more than one pair. Three may be ideal. You can't go wrong with a classic straight-leg in a higher waist-style in dark indigo. For a contrast, you could choose a softer, slightly faded pair in a casual bootleg. Then maybe a pair in another colour, such as black. We all have black trousers, but they tend to look far too formal; black denim works when black is called for but the occasion is more casual.

And if it's just going to be the one pair? A smart, straight-leg pair in a classic dark indigo colour with no deliberate fading (and no decoration, definitely no sequins!) will be a good investment. Team them with a tailored jacket, a luxurious knit, a summer coat or a wrap-dress, and they'll be worn time and time again.

## Jeans for all

✓ Feel your bottom half is still rather heavy? . . . Wide-leg styles are fashion winners, because they hide the legs, accentuate a slim waist and balance out the proportion of a wide shoulder or a larger bust. To further accentuate the slimming effect on top, a fitted shirt or blouse is called for – try a loose cardigan-style tunic to still hide, if you need to. However, a wide top with these wide bottoms will make you look like a cube, so only try wide-leg jeans if you're prepared to show the waistband and wear a belt!

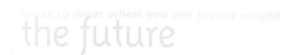

the future

✓ Legs too short? . . . Avoid flared styles, go for a straight or skinnier leg and check out petite ranges to save time on shortening the hem. (It's very hard to replicate the industrial stitching with your own sewing.)

✓ Tummy too round? . . . Look for a sophisticated side-zip fastening; it creates a super smooth tum and will be sufficiently high-waisted to smooth out any protrusion. Or buy a low-rise style, but wear a long top until it's safe to reveal all!

## Jeans dangers

✗ **Jeans too tight in the bum** . . . will pull around the groin area in front — very unflattering for us ladies.

✗ **Waistband too tight** . . . will reveal unflattering bulges of flesh, no matter how slim we are now.

✗ **Jeans too low** . . . who on earth thinks that a G-string, or indeed any underwear visible above the waistband, is attractive?

## Jeans made-to-measure

Jeans sizing is notoriously different from brand to brand. Try on as many pairs as you can — all frustrations will fly out of the window when you find the perfect pair! Some brands have recognised that are bums are different shapes and they offer different shapes in the equivalent of bra-cup-sizes A, B, C, etc. Other brands offer a fitting service and a bespoke make — the waiting time is usually around one month and the cost is approximately the price of a posh handbag. Depending on your location, you can find this kind of service in city-centre, big department stores. Once your details are stored on-site, you can re-order without returning to be fitted again.

Are you now of 'petite' proportions? So many brands and design ranges now carry petite ranges that you have as much choice as regular sizes. Look for neat, fitted styles that don't drown you. Fine, delicate details like embroidery, fine ruffles and lace trims will be perfect. Don't consider anything floor-length or you'll look like you're disappearing under all the fabric! For evening, choose 'cocktail'-length styles and heels. Keep accessories petite too.

## Top tops

Tops can help refine and define your shape, if you choose the right ones for you!

✓ If your arms and shoulders are still not what you'd like, try a tunic style like a kaftan — but not tent-shapes, which will do nothing for you. A floaty, slightly-transparent fabric with slight waist-shaping will add femininity. If the neckline is a deep V-shape or slit-shape, it will look sexy without being overtly so.

✓ To disguise the tummy area, choose a top which flares out from under the bust and skims over the stomach and hips. This will give emphasis to the top half of your body and below the waist – but only in a non-cling fabric like cotton or linen; anything too clingy will ruin the entire effect.

✓ To give the illusion of a fuller bust, and therefore a slimmer waist, choose a top with detail in the bust area – such as embellishment, ruching or a twist front – or a side wrap.

# A boost for bottoms

✓ **If you're an apple-shape** . . . try flat-fronted skirts and trousers – side-zips have the flattest fronts and consequently the most power to create the smoothest tum. Avoid pleats at all costs.

✓ **If you're a pear-shape** . . . try bottoms which emphasise the curves, but which have a slimming and lengthening effect as well. For instance, a pencil skirt or long tailored trousers (even a pinstripe), teamed with a tailored or shaped top which emphasises the bust. Avoid bottoms in any thin, clingy fabric, or bottoms with fancy detailing around the hips.

✓ **If you're evenly curvy** . . . choose bottoms which emphasise your waist and give equal attention to your bosom and hips. Tailoring wins hands down.

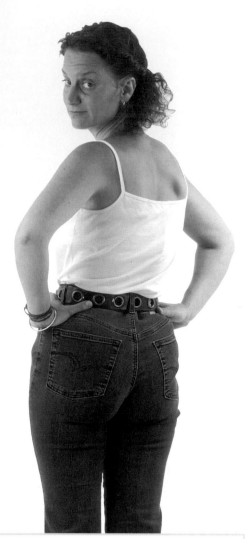

Don't tuck-in tight styles if you're a pear...
it just emphasises the roundness.

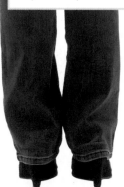

More fluid tailored styles elongate
the body – much more flattering!

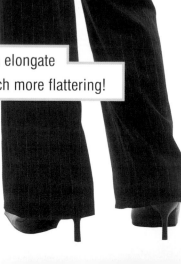

the future

# Dare we try a dress?

**Yes!** – particularly the wrap-dress or at least a crossover-top-style. With their deep V-neckline they draw attention away from the waist and yet manage to create the effect of having a cleavage too, particularly helpful if you've slimmed your bosom right down. And a dress doesn't have to be worn with tights or bare legs any more; dresses are trendy when worn over trousers or jeans and even leggings or footless tights these days – very useful for less-than-perfect legs.

## FACT

During our journey, some of us may have lost a bit more weight from our breasts than we actually wanted to. However, uplift, padded and gel-filled bras - and an invention comically known as the chicken fillet – can all work wonders to enhance what we have got left! Visit a good quality lingerie shop (many department stores have very good underwear departments too) and ask to be measured and fitted. Once you are happy with the feel of a bra, pop your top back on and look at your profile. A well-fitting bra should give you a perkier more uplifted look. Make sure you check the fit of the straps regularly.

## Dare we do print?

Print tops and plain bottoms help disguise a pear-shape and, in reverse, a plain top and patterned bottom will disguise a large bust. It's simple: patterns seek attention; people's eyes will be drawn to something bright and intricate, rather than plain. Just be wary of teaming prints with colourful matching accessories as this can look a little too much. Summer prints look fresh and fabulous teamed with white and denim. Winter rich patterns, like paisleys, look even more rich and gorgeous when teamed with autumnal fine-wool classics.

**FACT**

Have you uncovered an hourglass figure? Choose styles to emphasise your shoulders and hips, to make your waist even tinier. Wear wide cinched-in belts with wide-leg trousers. The wrap-dress was made for you, as well as all the 40s vintage styles. You're able to carry off the low cut top/cleavage look by being in perfect proportion to your hips. And you can make mannish tailoring look gorgeously feminine. Go for it!

the future

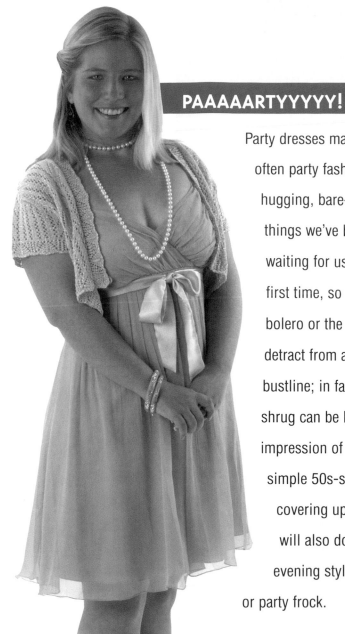

## PAAAAARTYYYYY!

Party dresses may have been off-limits to us until now, because often party fashion isn't designed without being bodice-hugging, bare-shouldered, sleeveless, halter-neck – all the things we've been desperate to avoid. Now, the dresses are waiting for us! It may take a little courage to wear one for the first time, so thank goodness for the re-introduction of the bolero or the shrug. This covers the shoulders but doesn't detract from a slim waistline because it fastens under the bustline; in fact, if your hips are still a little wide a bolero or shrug can be helpful to your overall proportion by giving the impression of a curvier top half. If you're still wary, try a simple 50s-style cardigan – this will do the same job of covering up arms, shoulders (and waist, if long enough). It will also double the opportunity of wearing a flimsy evening style, by turning it into a less formal, fun cocktail or party frock.

Party dresses are no longer off-limits and disguising problem areas is easy with boleros and wraps.

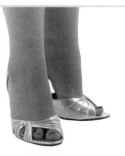

Colour is the most important statement you can make with evening wear. For winter (think Christmas and New Year celebrations), there are some shades that will always spell evening; predictable perhaps, but their longevity in this niche exists because it works – we're talking black, purples and plums, chocolate-browns and greys and bottle-greens. For summer (think weddings and May balls and garden party events), it really depends on the seasonal choice by your favoured designer, label or brand. For instance, if pink is 'in', you'll be pushed to find a favourite spring green. When choosing a colour, particularly for separates, try to choose tonal rather than clashing or opposing colours to make the look more coordinated and pulled together. Separates from different brands can look like one total 'designer' look just in the choice of complementary colour and fabrics.

Party and special occasion wear is really down to personal taste. Rather than worrying about what to wear, this time around you'll be spoiled for choice. For instance, our choice of trouser is much wider now; we can choose satin and shiny fabrics without being in danger of them looking taut and about to burst. The biggest worry you'll have now is if someone else turns up wearing what you're wearing! Enjoy this new dilemma . . .

Rather than worrying about what to wear, this time around you'll be spoiled for choice.

the future

What better instant fashion fix than a pair of sunglasses? For a relatively small outlay, a piece of 'eye-candy' can add an air of mystique and give off bags of confidence – even if you're not feeling it. Round faces need frames that are the same width or slightly wider than the fullest part of the face. High corners can help create a longer profile. Long faces need frames which are wider than their depth and a low bridge to make the nose look shorter. A design incorporating a decorative top will help by adding width. Square faces need curves to soften the angular look. Heart-shaped faces need detail or decoration running at the bottom of the frame, to make the lower face look wider. Don't forget that sunglasses add an air of style even if they're not on your face, but on the top of your head . . .

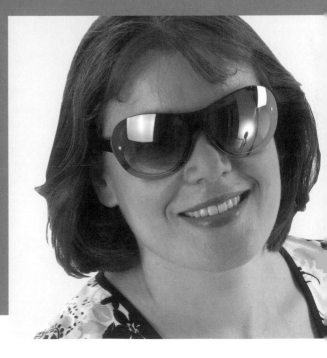

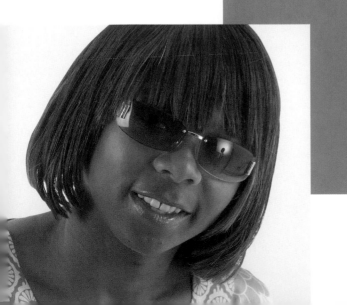

## The perfect swimsuit

At our heaviest, there were limited swimwear styles available – and they were often decidedly mumsy, to say the least. Now that our shapes are emerging like a butterfly from the proverbial chrysalis, it's interesting to learn the rules of swimsuit-buying – what, in theory, should suit our different figure types. Although, if you really want to go for that pink hibiscus print, wear it with pride!

If you don't feel ready for a bikini, a tankini is an ingenious and relatively new take on the two-piece

If you still want to hide your tummy, opt for a swimsuit with 'tummy control' and also good bust support – this will detract attention from the tummy area. Look at styles with an actual cup, or with concealed support. Now we have a pert bod, we don't want to be let down – 'down' being the operative word – with a less-than-pert bosom. These styles are perfect, too, for minimising a larger bust if you're conscious of being top-heavy. However, if your weight loss has left you with even less on top than you wanted to lose, smaller busts can take advantage of padded, moulded or gel-filled bra-styles; modern inventions are there to help us to even things up.

If you don't feel ready for a bikini, a tankini is an ingenious and relatively new take on the two-piece. A tankini consists of a vest-style top with pants,

the future

so it has the convenience of a two-piece bikini (bathroom breaks) and sunbathing potential (easy to roll up the top when you're lying flat), with the coverage of a one-piece. But do make sure that the length of the vest-top meets up with the pants, to avoid unslightly bulges of flesh around the midriff. You can often buy tankinis as separates, which helps to ensure a great fit if your top half and bottom half aren't the same size.

As for colours, it's true that darker shades are more slimming – there's a reason for the popularity of black and navy-blue swimwear. But now that we're nearly goal weight, don't be afraid to experiment with colours and patterns. As with day clothes, you can use colour and pattern to accentuate your best features, detract from features you're less happy with, and balance up your overall appearance. For instance, pear-shapes can emphasise the bust with a bright colour or patterned top half and a darker solid colour on the bottom, or with an uplifting underwired style to give cleavage and distraction.

One-piece dark swimsuits are universal design classics; the tankini is the next step up but only when you've said au-revoir to any 'overhang'!

When it comes to beach holidays, rather than swimming for exercise, don't forget that swimwear today doesn't stop at a one-piece or a two-piece. Designers now make short wrap-skirts, longer sarongs, and cover-all kaftans to match, so there's no reason not to feel comfortable when wandering from the pool to the sunlounger, and beyond. Covering up is also a sensible option if you're unsure of the SPF of your sunblock. Treat yourself and buy several pieces to create a whole swimwear wardrobe.

Nowadays, you can easily find fancy flip-flops with a small heel, to lengthen your leg, complement your outfit, and put some style into your walk. And sunhats, sunglasses, hairbands and clips, and even one or two pieces of carefully matched jewellery (earrings, bangles, ankle-bracelets) can all be used to focus people's attention away from bits you're always going to be conscious of, no matter how slim you are.

the future

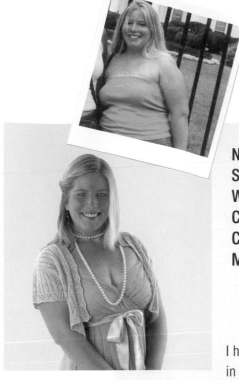

| | |
|---|---|
| **Name:** | Louise Green |
| **Start weight:** | 13 stone 6 pounds |
| **Weight now:** | 9 stone 10 pounds |
| **Clothes size before:** | 16 to 18 |
| **Clothes size now:** | 10 to 12 |
| **Meeting:** | Bognor Regis, Sussex |

I have always been described as curvy or chubby, and when kids in the street started to laugh and call me fat, I decided something had to be done about it. A few years before, I had lost over 19 pounds with Weight Watchers. I had let the weight creep back on, but now I was determined to lose it again – and more, and to change my lifestyle permanently.

Weight Watchers is the only diet plan that has ever worked for me. It is realistic, so I know I can stick to it. I used the NoCount plan, as my problem is not feeling full enough after a meal and then snacking – especially on crisps and cheese (which I cut out completely). I also did more exercise; I enjoy swimming and walking, and I did the Race for Life for Cancer Research. Seeing the pounds come off steadily kept me motivated: I reached my goal weight after six months but lost a few pounds extra – I wanted to give myself a bit of leeway. I cheered when I got into size 10 clothes for the first time! I have always loved clothes, but felt before that I could never wear certain items, such as skirts. Now I love showing off bits I couldn't reveal before.

The best thing about losing weight was a huge growth in my confidence. I received so many compliments from my family and friends, as well as the regular customers at the pub where I work part-time. I have graduated from my university Fine Art degree with a 2:1, and started work with the Youth Offending Service without having to worry all the time what people think of me. My fiancé is nice and thin and I always felt so ridiculously big compared to him – I am looking forward to getting married next year in whatever dress I like, and seeing us side by side in the photos.

# Success stories

**Name:** Fiona Andreanelli
**Start weight:** 9 stone 10 pounds
**Weight now:** 8 stone 7 pounds
**Weight lost:** 1 stone
**Clothes size before:** 12+
**Clothes size now:** 8 to 10
**Meeting:** Camberley, Surrey

I was always a small, skinny child, and became a petite adult – but with a very healthy appetite! From about age 20, I got a bit heavier every year. The turning point came when I was 31. I was in love, and very happy. Our house was being renovated, and we had been without a kitchen for two months, living on microwaveable ready-meals and takeaways. I was bigger than ever. My mother came round to fit a party-dress pattern template to me, and she had to cut one two sizes larger than usual! I was horrified – but I was even more horrified after the party, when I saw the photos in that dress. I realised my weight had spiralled out of control.

I joined Weight Watchers and followed the NoCount plan, as it was no-nonsense and there were plenty of ingredients on the list that I loved. Soon, I was dropping two pounds a week – and loving it! I began to cook up a frenzy in my new kitchen with the help of the Weight Watchers cookbooks. When I had friends over for dinner, they could never tell they were eating low-fat recipes.

I shot past my goal weight despite going on an all-inclusive holiday in the middle of my weight-loss plan! The old Fi would have eaten everything in the buffet, but I stayed disciplined and made sure I used the gym facilities. I love being able to see the bone structure of my face, to try on trousers without bursting into tears, and to wear shorts. I have inspired many of my thirty-something friends who are heavier than they would like, and am training to become a Weight Watchers leader myself.

**Fiona's style tip:** Make the most of your good bits and hide the bits you are less keen on.

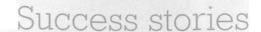

## Success stories

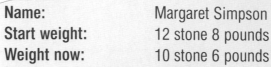

| | |
|---|---|
| **Name:** | Margaret Simpson |
| **Start weight:** | 12 stone 8 pounds |
| **Weight now:** | 10 stone 6 pounds |
| **Clothes size before:** | 18 to 20 |
| **Clothes size now:** | 12 to 14 |
| **Meeting:** | Winchester, Hampshire |

I knew I had to lose weight when – on top of feeling big, unfit and generally unwell – severe backache became a real problem, stopping me from doing what I wanted with my life. At first I tried to lose weight by dieting on my own – but with little success. I decided to join Weight Watchers, and got started at an evening meeting I could attend after work. My job was stressful, and after a long heavy day in the office, I usually rushed into the hall to get weighed but rarely stayed for the meeting afterwards. As the weight began to come off, I thought I could manage without attending even the weigh-ins. However, after four months trying to follow the weight-loss plan on my own, the weight was creeping on, rather than off!

When I gave up full-time employment, I decided to find a morning meeting instead. The style and atmosphere were unhurried and relaxed – and the difference this made to me was huge. I began to stay to the meetings and join in the group discussions. This helped me keep motivated and the weight started to come off once more.

Now I have reached goal weight, I am so much more active. I no longer need osteopathy sessions once a week, but am on a maintenance programme of one every six weeks. I am fit enough to do more exercise, and I feel and look great!

**Margaret's style tip:** If you are having trouble finding the right clothes because you are between sizes, then buy some nice accessories instead – they will update an outfit and add some colour and fun.

# Recipes for success

## Savoury or sweet — you can't go wrong with these low *POINT* recipes.

### Turkey ciabatta grills

1 ciabatta loaf with sun-dried tomatoes or olives

2 tablespoons sun-dried tomato paste

150 g (5¹/2 oz) grilled red and yellow pepper strips

8 medium turkey rashers, uncooked

salt and freshly ground black pepper

a few basil leaves

serves 4 — 4½ POINTS VALUE — Per serving — 225 cals

- Preparation and cooking time 10 minutes.
- Freezing not recommended.
- 18 *POINTS* values per recipe

Turkey rashers make a tasty topping.

1   Preheat the grill to high.

2   Slice the loaf in half lengthways and spread with the tomato paste.

3   Top both pieces of ciabatta with the pepper strips, then the uncooked turkey rashers. Grill for 1¹/2 minutes, then turn the rashers over and grill for another 1¹/2 minutes, until the rashers are cooked.

4   Slice each piece of bread in half, then serve, seasoned with salt and pepper and scattered with a few basil leaves.

**Cook's note:** Look for grilled pepper strips in jars, preserved in vinegar, then rinse and drain them. Alternatively, you can buy canned red peppers (sometimes called pimientos) which simply need to be drained and sliced.

**Variation:** Buy plain ciabatta loaves if you can't find ciabatta with sun-dried tomatoes or olives. The *POINTS* values per serving will be the same.

### Grilled lamb steaks with mint and lemon

2 x 150 g (5¹/2 oz) lamb leg steaks

1 tablespoon mint jelly

finely grated zest of 1 lemon

25 g (1 oz) fresh wholemeal breadcrumbs

15 g (¹/2 oz) fresh Parmesan cheese, grated

salt and freshly ground black pepper

serves 2 — 5½ POINTS VALUE — Per serving — 355 cals

- Preparation time 15 minutes.
- Cooking time 25 minutes.
- Freezing recommended.
- 11 *POINTS* values per recipe

1   Preheat the oven to Gas Mark 5/190˚C/375˚F. Line a baking tray with non-stick baking parchment.

2   Rinse the lamb steaks and pat dry with absorbent kitchen paper. Arrange on to the baking sheet.

3   Mix together the mint jelly, lemon zest, breadcrumbs, Parmesan and seasoning. Spread evenly over each steak.

4   Bake for 25 minutes until the lamb is cooked through.

# Tomato and basil platter

4 beef tomatoes, thinly sliced

12 baby plum or cherry tomatoes, halved

1 bunch of spring onions, trimmed and finely chopped

a handful of basil leaves, torn into shreds

salt and freshly ground black pepper

**For the dressing**

1 tablespoon olive oil

2 teaspoons lemon juice

1 garlic clove, chopped

serves 4 · ½ POINTS VALUE · Per serving · 75 cals · V

- Preparation time 10 minutes + 30 minutes standing time.
- Freezing not recommended.
- 2½ **POINTS** values per recipe

1   Arrange the beef tomatoes on to a large serving platter, fanning out the slices. Top with the plum or cherry tomato halves, then sprinkle with the spring onions.

2   Mix together the olive oil, lemon juice and garlic. Season with salt and pepper.

3   Sprinkle the dressing over the individual salads. Cover with clingfilm and leave at room temperature for about 30 minutes to allow time for the flavours to develop.

4   Serve, scattered with the basil leaves.

**Cook's note:** When all the different varieties of tomatoes are in season, it's a good idea to use them to make this fabulous salad.

# Spiced carrot and sultana salad

1 tablespoon sesame oil

½ tablespoon poppy seeds

1 teaspoon cumin seeds

15 g (½ oz) pine kernels

450 g (1 lb) carrots, peeled and coarsely grated

50 g (1¾ oz) raisins or sultanas

2 tablespoons seasoned rice vinegar

salt and freshly ground black pepper

serves 4 · 1½ POINTS VALUE · Per serving · 145 cals · V

- Preparation and cooking time 20 minutes.
- Freezing not recommended.
- 6 **POINTS** values per recipe

1   Heat the sesame oil in a large saucepan that has a lid. Add the poppy seeds and cumin seeds. Put the lid on and heat until the seeds start to pop. Take care that the seeds do not burn.

2   Remove the saucepan from the heat and add the pine kernels, stirring to mix.

3   Put the grated carrots into a serving bowl and add the seeds, nuts and any remaining oil. Add the raisins or sultanas and vinegar, then season with salt and pepper. Toss together well, then serve.

**Cook's note 1:** If you have a food processor, use it to make light work of grating the carrots.

**Cook's note 2:** This is an excellent dish for a buffet, served with a selection of other salads.

**Variation:** If you can't find seasoned rice vinegar, use white wine vinegar instead.

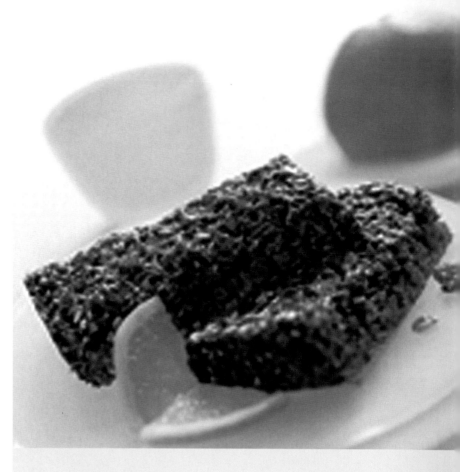

## Orange and sesame flapjacks

125 g (4¹/2 oz) butter
125 g (4¹/2 oz) demerara sugar
3 tablespoons golden syrup
finely grated zest of 1 orange
2 tablespoons sesame seeds
1 teaspoon ground cinnamon
225 g (8 oz) rolled oats

serves **8**  **7** POINTS VALUE®  Per serving **330** cals **V**

- Preparation time 15 minutes + 5 minutes cooling.
- Cooking time 20 minutes.
- Freezing not recommended.
- 54¹/2 **POINTS** values per recipe

1   Preheat the oven to Gas Mark 5/190°C/375°F. Line an 8-inch (20 cm) square cake tin with non-stick baking parchment.

2   Place the butter, sugar and syrup in a small saucepan and heat gently until dissolved.

3   Mix together the orange zest, sesame seeds, cinnamon and oats. Pour the melted butter mixture over and stir well. Press into the lined tin.

4   Bake for 20 minutes. Allow to cool.

# Peach brûlée

1 medium fresh, ripe peach or 2 canned peach halves

2 tablespoons low-fat plain yogurt

1 tablespoon golden granulated or demarara sugar

serves 1

2 POINTS VALUE · Per serving

105 cals

V

- Preparation and cooking time 5 minutes + cooling
- Cooking time 25 minutes.
- Freezing not recommended.
- 2 **POINTS** values per recipe

A very simple but tantalising pudding that you can make for yourself in just a few minutes.

1   Preheat the grill to high. Place the peaches in a shallow serving bowl or plate and spoon on the yogurt. Sprinkle over the sugar and grill until the sugar is melted. Cool for a minute or two until the sugar crisps up then serve.

**Variation:** Use virtually fat-free fromage frais instead of yogurt for 1¹/2 points per serving.

# Rhubarb and custard fool

900 g (2 lb) rhubarb, trimmed and cut into 5 cm (2-inch) lengths

100 g (3¹/2 oz) demarara sugar

zest of 1 orange

2 x 150 g pots ready-to-serve low fat cuslard

serves 4

2¹/2 POINTS VALUE · Per serving

165 cals

V

- Preparation and cooking time 20 minutes.
- Cooking time 20 minutes.
- Freezing not recommended.
- 9¹/2 **POINTS** values per recipe

An old-fashioned rhubarb fool is still a delicious way to round off a meal.

1   Put the rhubarb in a saucepan with the sugar, orange zest and 2 tablespoons of water. Cover and simmer over a gentle heat for 5 minutes or until just tender.

2   Drain, reserving a little of the liquid, and purée in a blender or put through a sieve. Add some of the cooking liquid if too thick but take care not to make it too wet. Set aside to cool.

3   Stir in the custard, pour into serving glasses and chill before serving.

# the end of the journey

D o you drive? Do you remember the mirror–signal–manoeuvre technique? Well, the journey you've been on for the past few months to a year, or even a little longer, started with that very same technique. First, you checked your mirror and decided things couldn't stay the same. Then, you signalled to the world and friends and family that things were going to change, and you outwardly made visible the different direction you were taking. Finally, you manoeuvred yourself into a totally different way of thinking and acting, to achieve what you've achieved. You made numerous positive lifestyle changes. Family and friends will have certainly noticed, perhaps even joined you on the journey without realising it.

Don't be downhearted if your journey wasn't simple. We may perhaps have got lost for a while along the way. We may have missed a turn we were supposed to take. We may have been diverted down an attractive scenic route, rather than following the more difficult route which led where we wanted to go. We perhaps sometimes felt caught in the slow lane, wondering if we would ever reach our destination. Of course, you got there in the end. And now, finally at your destination, you want to continue this worthwhile journey. You are committed to go on following your healthy lifestyle.

Now you're taking pleasure in your wonderful new wardrobe, it's important to remember a few key points. Always care for your clothes: check hems, sew loose buttons back on, have dry-cleanables dry-cleaned, always hang clothes on hangers – care for them and they will repay you with a longer life. Update core basics as soon as they show wear and tear. Replace whites regularly; white doesn't stay white for very long. Black also tends to fade; a new black looks much more chic than last year's used-to-be-black-now-charcoal-grey shade. Keep a check on trends and update styles if necessary – if you're not keen on splashing out on new garments, try adopting an 'in' colour as a scarf or bold piece of jewellery.

Sadly, as we humans don't possess an in-built satellite navigation system, there's no computer chip with a wealth of fashion knowledge and an automated voice telling us which direction to take every day. But we have something better, something that all computers were designed to resemble – our brains. We have done the preparation – now the fashion world is ours to plunder.

# the end of the road

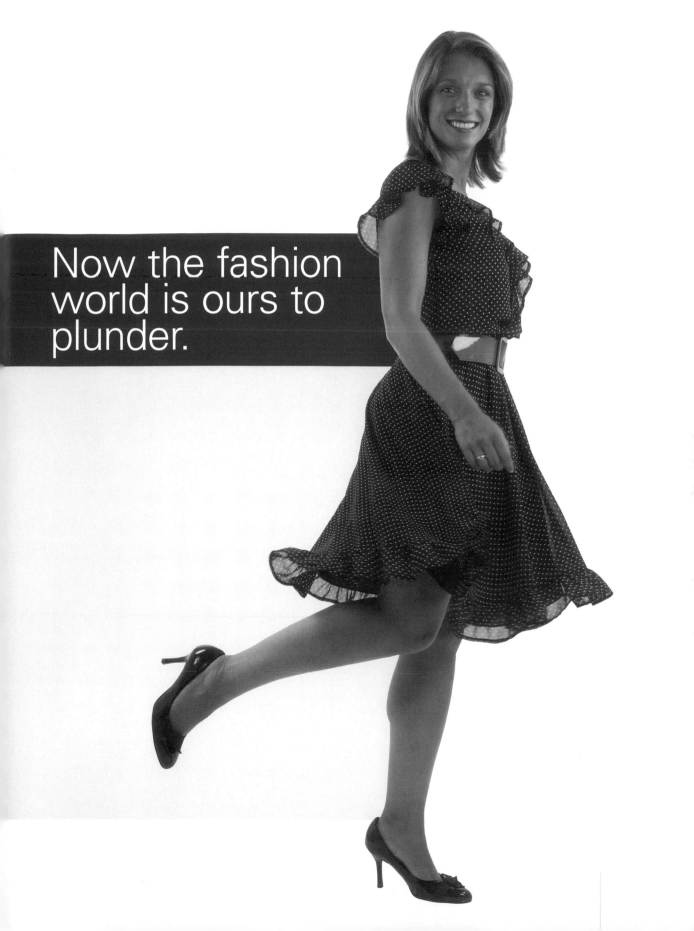

Now the fashion
world is ours to
plunder.

address book

address book addre

## Ann Harvey

Over 100 stores in the UK. Casual and special occasion clothes in sizes 16 to 28. Medium-price range.

Tel: 01582 399877

## Anna Scholz

Perhaps the only designer actively designing a collection aimed specifically at the larger market. Interestingly, her clothes are graded down to regular sizes! Up to size 26. Available Harrods and Selfridges, London. Diffusion range available within Simply Be. Catalogues available – 0870 6068000

Tel: 0208 964 3040   www.annasholz.com

## Bravissimo

Bravissimo is a company that provides a wide choice of lingerie and swimwear in D to JJ cups, as well as clothing designed especially for big-boobed women. Mail order, 12 high-street stores, and online.

Tel: 01926 459 859   www.bravissimo.com

## Bon Marche

Affordable fast-fashion styles from regular sizes up to size 24. 360 stores nationwide.

Tel: 01924 700100   www.bonmarche.co.uk

address book

## Chesca

Luxury soft tailoring and knits, day and evening wear and special occasion wear in sizes 14 to 24. Over 30 concessions within major department stores throughout the UK and online.

Tel: 0207 6093434   www.chesca1424.co.uk

## Debenhams

120 stores in major cities nationwide. Debenhams' own 'Collection' range (slightly more mature styling) is available up to size 20.

Tel: 08456 055044   www.debenhams.com

## Elvi Sizes

Casual and evening styles in sizes 16 to 26. Mid-price range. 90 UK outlets, some stand-alone stores, others, concessions within department stores.

Tel: 01527 506 306   www.elvi.co.uk

## Emotion

Makers of wide-fitting women's footwear and boots (E–EEE fittings).

Tel: 01642 807090   www.emotionshoes.co.uk

## www.eplussizeclothes.com

Website devoted to plus-sized market in sizes 18 to 42.

Tel: 01670 524150

## Evans

Affordable to mid-price range daywear and casual separates. Young through to mature styles in sizes 16 to 32. Style consultants available in 20 stores. Underwear sizes 38" to 50", cup sizes B–H – all stores offer a bra measuring and fitting service. Footwear in wider fittings, size 4 to 10. Tall range available for over 5'10" and petite range for 5'2" and under.

Customer Enquiries: 0845 121 4516   www.evans.co.uk

## Fenwick Ltd (Brent Cross)

Plus-size department with up to fifteen different fashion labels, offering daywear to cruise to eveningwear, and dedicated to sizes 18 to 26. Mid-to high-price range in good quality fabrics. Brands include Frankenwalder and Gerry Weber.

Tel: 0208 202 8200   www.fenwick.co.uk

## Figleaves.com

The world's largest online retailer of branded 'intimates' including lingerie, swimwear and sleepwear in average sizes. Best supplier of 'control' underwear including Spanx Power panties, Spanx hide and sleek panties, Miraclesuit, Magic knickers, Magic Slimshot, Rago Waist Cinch, Rago padded shaper panty, Flexees by Maidenform waistshaper brief, Sassybax, Falke shaping shorts, and Falke 20, denier shaping control tights.

Tel: 0870 499 9000   www.figleaves.com

## Harrods

The Plus Collections department caters for sizes 18 to 28; high-end designer collections in luxury fabrics. Currently stocking Almia, Anna Scholz, Basler, James Lakeland, Elena Miro, Marina Rinaldi (and Sport), Gian Franco Ferre, Persona, Wille, Quintess, Eileen Fisher, Charles and Patricia Lester, Bione Fragola and Harrods Capes.

87–135 Brompton Road, London SW1X 7XL Tel: 0207 730 1234 www.harrods.com

## H&M

The Big is Beautiful range is in 43 out of 103 UK stores. Affordable cotton and jersey mix pieces in trendy younger styles. UK sizing is 16 to 30 but described as medium for sizes 14 to 16; large for sizes 18 to 20; XL for sizes 22 to 24; 2XL for sizes 26 to 28 and 3XL for size 30.

Tel: 0207 323 2211   www.hm.com

## Lands End

Regular sizing in most styles up to sizes 20 to 22, some styles available in 2X (sizes 24 to 26) and limited styles in 3X (28 to 30). They say 'instead of adding centimetres of fabric on to smaller sizes, our products are re-proportioned for a fantastic fit to flatter the fuller figure'.

Tel: 0800 3767974   www.landsend.co.uk

## La Redoute

One of the best mail order selections of the season's trends. Affordable to mid-price ranges. Most items available up to size 20, selected styles up to 22 and specialist collections up to size 24.

0870 0500 455   www.laredoute.co.uk

## LXdirect

Affordable casual selected styles up to size 28. Other styles available in sizes 8 to 22.

Tel: 0845 7573457   www.lxdirect.com

## Long Tall Sally

29 stores nationwide. Specific 'longer in the body' casual and tailored smart separates and special occasion wear for tall girls who require 34" and 36" leg lengths and longer sleeve lengths; many of the styles are

address book

available in size 20, others in up to size 18.

Mail order 0870 990 6885   www.longtallsally.com

## Marina Rinaldi and Marina Sport

Premium quality tailoring, evening wear and luxury casual in sizes 14 to 26 Flagship stores in Bond St, London, and Edinburgh.

Head office tel: 0207 580 5075

## M&S

Plus-range of medium-priced casual and special occasion (more mature) styles in sizes 20 to 28 in approximately 65 main stores out of the overall 400 stores nationwide and online.

Tel: 0845 302 1234   www.marksandspencer.com

## Next and Next Directory mail order

Nationwide high-street fashion store, medium-priced range and affordable tailoring and casual styles. Good quality make and better than average fabrics. Selected styles up to size 22 and selected style wide-fitting shoes too.

Tel: 0845 600 7000   www.next.co.uk

## Penny Plain

Mid-price range full wardrobe selection of soft tailoring through to holiday styles in high-quality fabrics. Sizes 10 to 26.

Tel: 0870 111 8180   www.pennyplain.co.uk

## Selfridges

Women's Casual Department houses sizes 16 to 26 (and some selected styles in size 28) from Marina Rinaldi, Persona, Quintesse by Frank Usher and Anna Scholz. Nearby DKNY Pure goes up to size 18 and there are generously cut pieces in the 18/20 size range from Shirin Guild and Oska.

General enquiries, Tel: 0870 837 7377; Women's casual department, Tel: 0207 318 3304   www.selfridges.com

## Sew Today

Monthly magazine devoted to home-sewing and the latest fashion patterns available from Vogue, McCalls and Butterick.

0870 777 9966   www.sewdirect.com

## Simply Be

On-trend online and home shop clothing range for the plus-size market in sizes 14 to 32 with selected sizes up to size 36. Affordable and mid-price range. Also designer range by Anna Scholz. Footwear to size 9.

Tel: 0870 1606100   www.simplybe.co.uk

## Sixteentwentysix by Florence + Fred at larger Tesco Extra stores

Casual affordable range in sizes 16 to 26.

Tel: 0800 505555   www.tesco.com/clothing

## Spirito Di Artigiano mail order

Luxury fabrics, classic styling, formal tailoring, special party pieces in sizes 16 to 30. Tel: 01983 531000   www.spirito.co.uk

## Tristan Webber Digital Couture (bespoke jeans)

In conjunction with the Bodymetrics light scanning measuring service.

Tel: 0870 086 9059

## Yours

Affordable casual styles plus lingerie and accessories. 40 stores in the Suffolk/Norfolk/Northampton/Leicestershire/Essex/Cambridgeshire and Bedfordshire areas and on line at www.yoursclothing.co.uk

Tel: 0800 0856540

# Index